# YOGA

## AND DIET FOR AILMENTS

# YOGA

## AND DIET FOR AILMENTS

BIJOYLAXMI HOTA

RUPA

Thanks to
Swami Swaroopanansa Saraswati (Bhubaneshwar) for teaching me yoga and helping me out whenever I have needed it.
My family P.C. Hota, Reema Singh, Prasenjit Hota, Reela Hota, Dhoopa Singh & Ishaan Hota for their invaluable inputs and unconditional support at every step.

*Published by*
Rupa Publications India Pvt. Ltd 2015
7/16, Ansari Road, Daryaganj
New Delhi 110002

*Sales centres:*
Allahabad Bengaluru Chennai
Hyderabad Jaipur Kathmandu
Kolkata Mumbai

ISBN: 978-81-291- 3496-7

First impression 2015
10 9 8 7 6 5 4 3 2 1

Designed by Ishtihaar.com, 91-11-2373 3200

Printed at Rakmo Press Pvt. Ltd., New Delhi

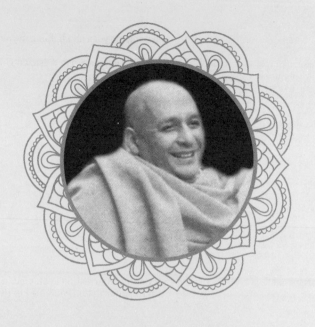

*With the blessings
of my Guru and Guide*

*Paramahamsa Swami Sri
Satyananda Saraswati*

# Contents

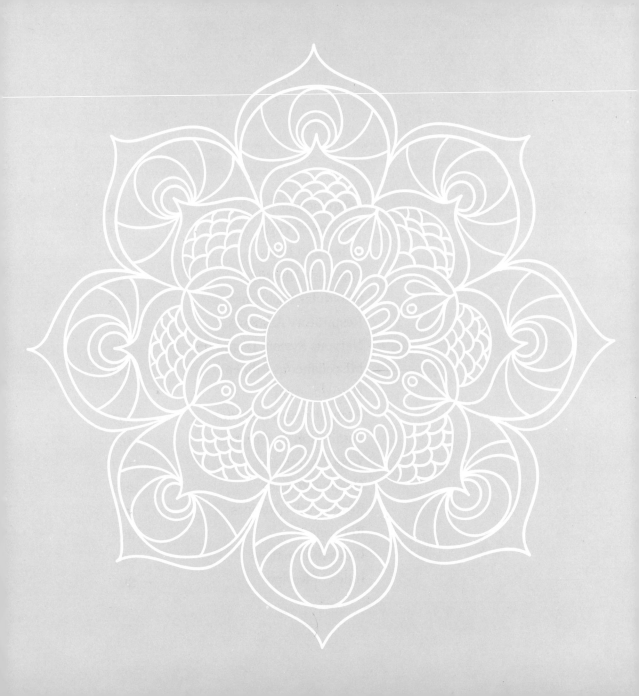

# Introduction

Yoga had cured me of ailments which had not responded to the other popular therapies. I practised it religiously, read and spoke about it, and in due course became a yoga therapist. I was getting very good results, but initially had not developed full confidence in the system. At this juncture, a gentleman came with multiple sclerosis. He had already deteriorated a lot and was unable to climb steps or rise from a sitting position without help. I wasn't too sure that yoga would help him, but seeing the hope in his eyes, I thought of giving it a try.

By then, I had developed my own style of Yogic treatment, where diet played a major role. I had realized early in my career that without appropriate diet a disease cannot be cured and yet no system had made full use of it. They all had different views of the subject, and although valid, their views were incomplete. For modern science, diet is vitamins and minerals, while Ayurveda regards it is mucus producing, gas producing and so on; and many other traditional therapies label it as just cooling or heating. And then there is the alkalinity and acidity factor which is very important but is completely overlooked by most therapists.

As my interest in health had led me to innumerable books on Nutrition, Ayurveda, Nature cure, and other therapies, I noticed this shortcoming and synthesized the different disciplines to get a complete and powerful guide to attain and maintain good health. When I added that to yoga the result was astounding. So I tried my new integrated therapeutic formula on this gentleman and to my utter relief and satisfaction, it worked. He started improving and by the end of the course of two months, he could do everything on his own. And the last time I heard of him—which was more than two decades from the day he came to me first—he was still mobile and fine.

Since then I have treated a wide variety of serious diseases. Initially, every time I encountered a new serious case, I used to feel quite unsure and apprehensive, but mercifully, the treatment never failed. Sometimes the cure might not have been total, either because of the advanced age of the patient or because of irreparable damage of his or her body part, but the improvement has always been there.

People who have experienced the efficacy of Integrated Yoga have developed an unshakable faith in this system. Twenty years ago, a doctor pronounced a wheezing two-year-old child as asthmatic and went on to describe its distressing prognosis to the young mother in great detail. The woman heard it all, faced the doctor squarely and said 'Doctor, six years hence you will see my child with no trace of asthma. I guarantee you that.' She asked for 'six years' because she knew that, a child could not practise yoga before the age of seven. Fortunately, she did not have to wait that long. With some natural remedies, and certain yogic practises meant for the mind—which I simplified for the baby—the child never wheezed again.

Incidents such as the above mentioned one gave me the confidence and encouragement to experiment, and the result has always been good. In this book I have tried to impart all my knowledge on health that I have gathered over more than thirty years as an Integrated Yoga therapist. If I have left out some ailments, it is because, either I did not get a chance to treat them, or have covered them in my previous books.

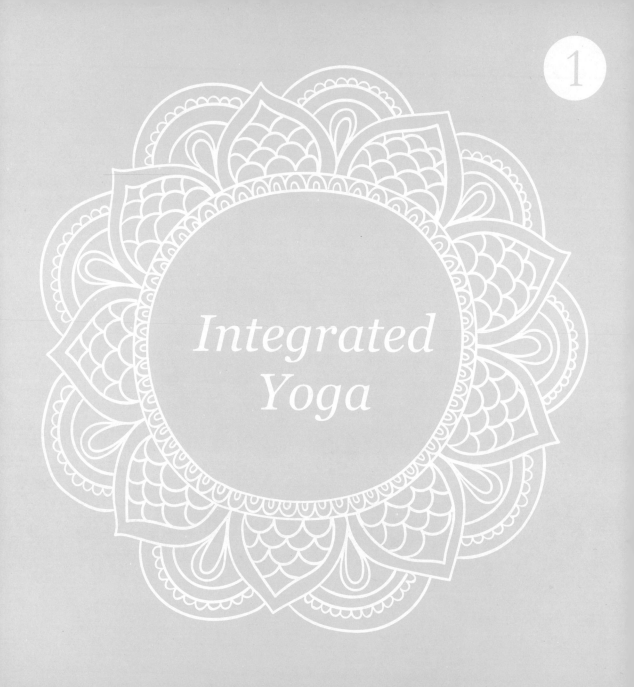

# Integrated Yoga

# 1

Medical science treats a disease according to its manifested symptoms. Ayurveda goes a little beyond that, and aims to pacify the humors. Some other therapies such as Acupuncture and Acupressure go still deeper and try to normalize the disturbed energy. All these health systems work on the physical aspects of a human being. But a disease is not always purely physical.

A human body is a complex mechanism that has a body, Prana, mind and a soul. And the mind itself has three different levels- conscious, subconscious and unconscious. A disease can start from any of the various aspects of an individual. In fact according to modern science, more than ninety percent of the diseases originate from the mind.

As mind is the mainspring of a disease, treating the body alone can not cure the affliction. It may suppress the symptoms for a while, but the cause of the disease remains which invariably brings back ill health - either as the same disease or a different one. Worst are therapies with medicines full of chemicals which add more poison to the already toxic and weak system making way for more serious ailments in future. At the same time, treating the mind alone does have not much value, as every tissue in the body is already affected adversely. They may not even have the strength to respond to the treatment.

Therefore to cure a disease, a system is needed that can recognize the fault and also has means to repair it. Integrated Yoga is such a system. It is the only therapy that has the techniques to counter each disease-causing factor and for that, it integrates practises from various yogas such as Hatha yoga, Raja yoga, Bhakti yoga, Mantra yoga, Tantra yoga etc.

# THE PRACTICES

## Asanas

Yogic postures are called asanas. With their stretching, flexing and twisting movements, these exercises squeeze the toxins out of the tissues, which are then carried out by the blood to be eliminated. They also draw a rich supply of blood to a target body part wherein the posture is held for a while for the blood to do the healing. Specific asanas affect specific parts of the body, and there are asanas to reach even the innermost ones.

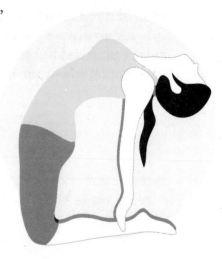

On the subtle level, asanas clear the energy pathways of pranic blockages so that prana—the vital life force—can flow freely in them. Prana, like blood is a major healing agent.

## Pranayama

These are breathing techniques that bring the external prana into the body to vitalize each tissue. This energy is first stored in energy centers called chakras and then distributed as, when and where it is needed. Pranayamas need asanas to precede them, to ensure that the paths are cleared before the energy is brought in to ply in them.

## Mudra

Having an abundance of prana in the chakras does not guarantee a cure. The energy has to reach the specific body part for the healing to begin. The job to channelize prana in the required direction is done by specific hand and body gestures called mudras. Pranayamas must be practised before or with mudras so that plentiful energy can be sent to the target area.

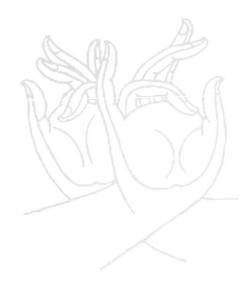

## Bandha

As the human body is a mass of swirling energy and not a solid structure, the stored prana leaks out continuously. To keep it within the body frame for a longer time, energy locks need to be created, which is done by various postures called bandhas.

## Satkarmas

Toxins in the system are a great hindrance for any cure. Unless they are removed first, practising yoga may not provide any benefit as the energy generated through asanas and pranayamas will be used up to eliminate these toxins and not for actual healing. It is because the body views toxins as life threatening and uses all the energy it can gather to expel them.

In hatha yoga, there are six purifying practises—neti, dhauti, basti,nauli, tratak and kapalbhati. Of them all, nauli and basti are the most difficult and can be skipped. The other four are very important. Dhauti washes the digestive tract while neti clears the nasal passage—both are extremely beneficial in today's highly polluted world. The last two practises are meant to energize the brain and clear unwanted elements from it.

## Yoganidra

The body heals best at night during deep sleep that consists of four phases—alpha, beta, theta and delta. Each of these stages has its own important functions. With tension and sleep medication, the phases are disturbed and even bypassed which diminishes the tissue rejuvenation capacity of the body. The tissues are only partially repaired and inadequately rested. Yoganidra is a technique, developed by my guru, the great yogi Paramahamsa Swami Satyananda Saraswati. It ensures sleep with all the four stages in the most ideal proportion which repairs the wear and tear of the body perfectly and facilitates a relaxed feeling that is most unique and pleasant.

## Meditation

Sometimes an extremely negative experience can cause a deep-rooted psychological impression which cannot be eliminated easily but through deep meditation. There are many kinds of meditation in the world. Though they all are equally effective, for the person to benefit properly, the method should be chosen according to individual need. For the best result, meditation should be followed by yoganidra.

## Bhajan

A person unhappy due to a personal tragedy may not benefit much from the normal yogic meditation. Rather, the more the person tries to take the mind inward, the more unhappy he or she becomes, as it helps keep the memories of the tragic experience fresh. For such people, bhajan (devotional music) belonging to nada yoga acts like a balm. Not only does the lilting music soothe frayed nerves, it also takes the mind away from the hurtful memories, giving it a chance to heal. Also, devotion itself is a great healer. It generates a strong positive emotion that overpowers all other emotions including the offending ones.

## Kirtan

This too is devotional music, belonging to nada yoga, but here, the names of the Supreme are repeated, and these names are said to be mantras with great healing powers. Used in yogic treatment for certain mental conditions, kirtan has yielded great results.

## Mantra

If a disease refuses to respond even to the best of yogic routines, it is thought to be 'karmic', i.e., the result of a negative deed which the sufferer is supposed to have done in this or a previous birth. It is believed that karmic result cannot be changed ordinarily but there are certain ways to do that—mantras being one of them. In yoga therapy, some

*Yoga and Diet for Ailments*

universal mantras and the bija mantras (core sound) of the chakras are used to treat karmic ailments and enhance healing.

· · · · · · · · · · · · · · · · · · · · · · · · · · · · · · · · · · · · · · · · · · · · · · · · · · · · · · · · · · ·

# THE ACCESSORIES

Yoga practises call for the following aids:

## Yoga Spread

Yoga needs a completely relaxed body to push the blood through the extremely thin blood capillaries. The muscles at the back loosen their grip and relax only when they feel a firm support from beneath. Traditionally, animal skin was used for yoga practises as its thickness and firmness were right for the body to relax. Also, animal skin produces electromagnetic waves that are health promoting. Next to animal skin, the best yoga spread is a pure wool blanket or rug. It is natural, thick and firm and still possesses some animal magnetism. Soft and spongy yoga mats should be avoided, especially if they are made from synthetic fabric, as that can decrease body's reserve energy.

## Yoga Dress

During yoga practise, the skin absorbs the atmospheric prana and oxygen. For that reason, it is necessary to wear loose and porous cotton clothing.

## Recorded Yoganidra

Although a live voice reciting yoganidra is most relaxing, that may not always be possible. A recorded yoganidra is a good substitute. Practising it on one's own is not very effective as the recollection of it keeps the brain active, whereas one needs a passive brain for complete relaxation. However, recorded meditation should be avoided as much as possible, because listening to a voice externalizes the mind. On the other hand meditation, unlike yoganidra, requires one to internalize it and be alert at the same time, to concentrate well. One can follow a recorded meditation only in the beginning in order to learn it.

## Mantra Mala (rosary)

Malas are essential for certain mantra repetition. There are different kinds of malas for different mantras. Rudraksh is generally used for most mantras. A combination of rudraksh and crystals is also highly regarded, as the male (positive) and female (negative) energies generated respectively by them, complement each other and produce an energy field which has a beneficial effect on the holder. Coloured stones used in conjunction with rudraksh are still better as these stones further stimulate the chakras having petals of corresponding colours.

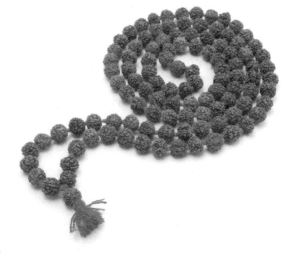

## Neti Pot

This is an invaluable object necessary for neti, a practise that clears the nose and facilitates better oxygenation of the system. It helps cure most respiratory and nervous system ailments. Only a natural metal or ceramic pot should be used for this practise. Artificial pots made of plastic are considered unhealthy.

## Arm rest

During mantra repetition, the right arm holding the mala must be kept away from the body to free the armpit of any obstructions because it is via this body part that the energy moves and even a slight pressure can disrupt the flow. In a long mantra meditation, keeping the arm in the required position for the entire duration can be tiring. A meditation armrest that yogis have been using since antiquity is a great help.

# RULES FOR PRACTISING YOGA

- Practise yoga on an empty stomach, i.e., either in the morning before breakfast or 3 to 4 hours after a meal
- Some food should be taken 20 minutes after practising yoga
- Yoga should not be done during fever and during the first four days of the menstrual cycle
- Terminate yoga practise if pain or discomfort is experienced during an asana
- Face east while practising yoga
- When you lie down in shavasana, the head should point towards the east

- If there is an urge to evacuate the bowel or bladder during yoga practise, it should not be ignored
- Breathe only through the nose unless a particular practise needs mouth breathing
- Fix a time for meditation and stick to it everyday
- If you are doing yoganidra once, it should be at bedtime
- Though twice a week is sufficient for general fitness, yoga should be practised more often to cure an ailment. Ideally, asanas, pranayamas, mudras and bandhas should be practised 5 days a week. One day should be kept for satkarmas. Once a week can be taken off from all yogic practices
- Meditation and yoganidra should be practised every day

If you have high blood pressure, first normalize it before tackling other problems.
The book **Yoga for a Healthy Heart** by the author contains how to do that in a week.

*Yoga and Diet for Ailments*

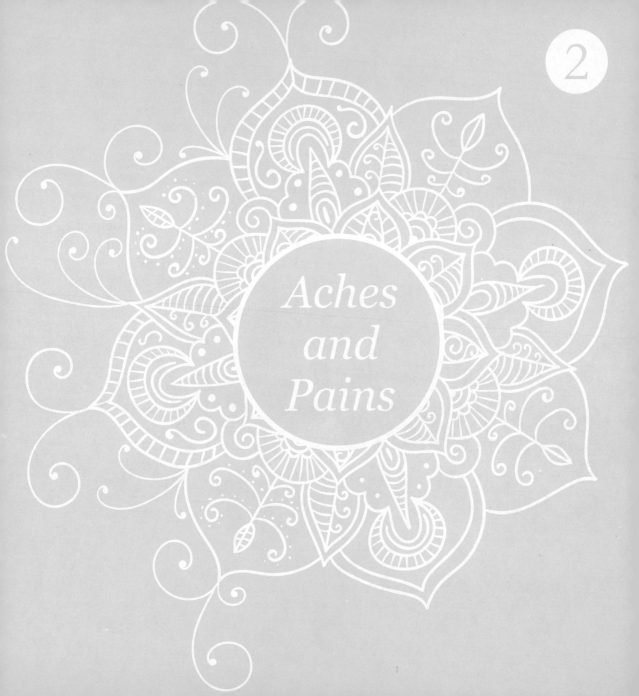

2

Aches
and
Pains

Pain is nature's way of drawing attention to a troubled body part for rectification. The discomfort should never be ignored as the problem could only worsen with time. Neither should it be suppressed with painkillers as their side effects can be far worse than the ailment itself. The reason for a pain must be determined at the first sign and removed as early as possible, as it is always more difficult to cure a chronic ailment.

# ARTHRITIS

**(Degenerative Osteoarthritis)**

## What

Inflammation of the joints due to friction of dry bones as the lubricant fluid dries up

## Why

- Injury to the joint that has not been rested enough to heal

- Rich acidic food that irritates the joint tissues

- Deficiencies of nutrients needed to make healthy joints, especially calcium, and Vitamins C and D

- Malfunctioning digestive system where nutrients required by the joint tissues are not absorbed and utilized

- Degeneration of the joints due to aging in an unhealthy body

- Excessive use of the joints as athletes do

- Stress as it interferes with the smooth functioning of the body

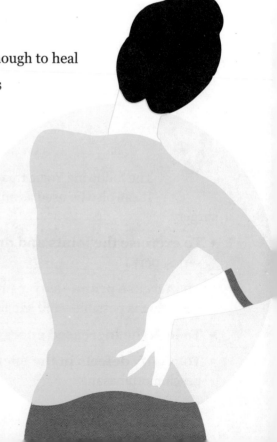

*Yoga and Diet for Ailments*

It occurs with pain in the joints—generally the weight-bearing ones such as the knees and hips—during and after use, and during season change. If left untreated, the joints are irreversibly damaged. The most conventional treatments are painkillers and surgery. Painkillers have many unpleasant side effects (see page 145) while surgery can lead to complications like:

- Formation of blood clots that can travel to the heart and lungs causing life threatening conditions such as heart attack and stroke

- Post-surgery infection which might require weeks of antibiotic treatment

- Contraction of the scar, leading to stiffness of the joint

- The ultimate wear and tear of the implant leading to its loosening and calling for corrective surgery, which is far more complicated

## Yogic Treatment

The following Yogic treatment can control arthritis in the initial stages. It can also be used as an effective method to counter the ill-effects of surgery.

- **To exercise the joints and draw prana to them**—pawanmuktasana series, part 1

- **To increase prana**—suryanamaskara—either the complete exercise or any steps that is possible—and kapalbhati pranayama

- **To lock the increased energy in the body**—maha bandha

- **To rectify defects in the energy field**—bhujangasana, dhanurasana, paschimottanasana

- **To clear the energy channels**—nadisodhan pranayama

- **To energize the bigger joints**—garudasana and vatayanasana

- **To de-stress the mind while normalizing chakra functions**—all chakra meditation

- **For rest and the best repair of worn-out tissues**—yoganidra at bedtime

- **Optional addition for faster healing**—single chakra meditation: on manipur chakra

## Role of food

Medicine in the form of food in the initial stage plays an equally vital role in the treatment of pain and the benefit from the following recipe of vegetable juice can help alleviate the symptoms of pain

**Recipe:** Extract the juice of—

1 raw potato

1 small bunch of spinach leaves

2 carrots

Mix them and drink it in the morning on an empty stomach

In the later stage, but before the cartilages are damaged, the following recipe for fenugreek tea can help with the symptoms.

**Recipe:** Boil 1 tsp of fenugreek seeds in a glass of water till the quantity is reduced to half. Add a pinch of turmeric powder and a pinch of salt, and drink it twice daily—first thing in the morning and at bedtime.

You will witness dramatic improvement within a month.

In the advanced stage organ therapy is said to be very effective. One needs to take animal cartilage in soup form.

The other beneficial kinds of food that provide relief are as follows:

- **Molasses**—often relief is felt within half an hour
- **Wheat germ oil**—helps in the regeneration process
- **Fish**—it has omega-3 that promotes the production of prostaglandin which brings down inflammation, and zinc that neutralizes the damaging effect of copper—a cause for this disease
- **Cod liver oil**—it lubricates the joints. The advantage of this medicine is that it goes directly to the joints, and not via the liver to be processed
- **Flax seed oil**—contains omega-3
- **Alfalfa and cabbage**—contain sulfur, the deficiency of which is also a cause of arthritis. Also, this mineral is a detoxifying agent
- **Honey**—it contains manganese, necessary for the joint tissues repair
- **Rose hip**—it is the richest source of Vitamin C; patients of arthritis need this vitamin in higher doses.
- **Turmeric**—it increases joint flexibility

As calcium and phosphorus are bone-forming minerals, food containing them should be focused on.

At the same time it is important to avoid food which is high in acid.
(see page 263)

# ARTHRITIS
## (inflammatory, i.e., rheumatoid arthritis)

### What

The body's immune cells attack the joint tissues and cause the inflammation

### Why

- Presence of bacteria or virus
- Nutritional deficiencies, especially of Vitamin A and pantothenic acid
- Lack of certain enzymes leading to undigested proteins which get into the joint tissues and are taken as harmful foreign matter by the immune cells to be attacked
- Permeable intestinal wall through which undigested food travels to the joints
- Acidic blood that irritates the joint tissues
- Stress, as it interferes with the smooth functioning of the system
- Constant irritability which leads to more acid secretion

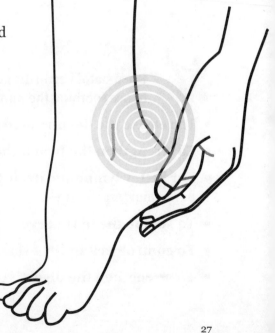

## Symptoms & conventional treatment

It occurs with pain and swelling in joints—mainly on the smaller ones such as the toes and fingers. There is a symmetrical appearance of symptoms and pain is more pronounced after a period of rest or inaction. The symptoms often come and go. However if left untreated, it can affect all the joints and turn the patient completely cripple. The most conventional form of treatment are anti-inflammatory drugs, and in severe cases, corticosteroids. However the side effects of anti-inflammatory drugs can cause nausea, vomiting, diarrhoea, constipation, loss of appetite, rashes, dizziness, drowsiness, headache, water retention, kidney failure, liver malfunction, ulcer, and prolonged bleeding after injury or surgery (for more, see page 146). Steroids can further cause glaucoma, cataract, high blood pressure, diabetes, obesity, osteoporosis, liver damage, testicular atrophy, and heart diseases.

## Yogic Treatment

Rheumatoid arthritis generally strikes after a traumatic experience; hence soothing the mind is very important in this ailment.

- **To release the deep-rooted stress**—cathartic meditation

- **To strengthen the heart, the emotional center**—hriday mudra

- **For better lymphatic drainage and to exercise all the joints**—part 1 of pawanmuktasana series

- **To soothe the taut nerves**—chant om 27 times and bhramari pranayama

- **To control irritability**—shashankasana—10 to 30 minutes

- **To strengthen the digestive system**—part 2 of pawanmuktasana series, paschimottanasana, dhanurasana and uddiyana bandha. Vajrasana should be done after meals

- **To clear the energy pathways**—nadisodhan pranayama
- **To promote natural steroid cortisone secretion**—akarna dhanurasan, ushtrasana
- **To burn body toxins**—bhastrika pranayama
- **For the best repair of the body tissues**—yoganidra at bedtime
- **To remove the excess acid and toxins from the system**—guru shankh prakshyalana. If unable to do this kriya—laghoo shankhaprakshyalan can be done daily for 45 days. Salt should be used only once or twice a week. If that kriya is also not possible, then one can follow other detoxifying methods (see page 134)
- **Optional addition for faster healing**—single chakra meditation on swadhisthana chakra

## Role of food

- **Amaltas leaves**—it repairs the damaged intestine. It should be ground and an amla (Indian gooseberry) size ball of the paste should be taken with half a cup of warm water in the morning on an empty stomach and 30 minutes after doing kunjal
- **Roasted coriander and cumin seeds (in proportion of 50:50)**—half a tsp thrice daily. It too repairs the intestine
- **Green juice**—extracted from wheat grass, barley grass, celery, basil and wood apple leaves. A strong alkaline, it neutralizes the content of the digestive tract and heals it

- **Rose hip**—it is the richest source of Vitamin C which increases immunity
- **Pro-biotic**—to kill the offending bacteria
- **Soya, fish and nuts**—they contain pantothenic acid which alleviates arthritic pain
- **Sweet fruits**—such as apple, papaya, musk melon
- **Bel (wood apple)**—tones up the liver and kills certain pathogens, especially amebiasis, which weakens the liver
- **Celery and grape juice**—are seen to give very good results
- **Garlic**—for its anti-inflammatory and anti-viral properties
- **Yeast**—rich in Vitamin B-complex that improves digestion and has nucleic acid which is essential for healthy cell formation
- **Turmeric**—to improve joint flexibility

Diet is the most important part in the treatment of this type of arthritis. As the system is acidic in this disease, the food must be highly alkaline. Secondly, the quantity of meals must be reduced to half. The number of meals may be increased if needed.

At the same time it is important to avoid sour and acid-forming food, (see page 263) as even a drop of citrus fruit juice can aggravate the pain. Green vegetables must be eaten in moderation. It is important to keep in mind that the stomach must never be filled, as the pain comes back almost immediately if it is full. Fasting once a week for 24 hours, i.e., missing any two consecutive meals is extremely beneficial in many ways, including reduced intestinal permeability.

For faster healing single chakra meditation on manipura can be done.

Reconstruction meditation also helps.

# BODY ACHE AND GROWING PAIN

## What

Discomfort that feels better when pressed

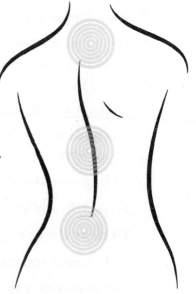

## Why

- Too many physical activities which tire the tissues and cause a dull, throbbing ache

- Lack of finer inner adjustments during growing up, causing severe pain in the limbs of youngsters

- Stress, as it disturbs the smooth functioning of the body

- Excessive uric acid in the blood

- Nutritional deficiencies, especially of calcium and Vitamin D

- Osteoporosis

- Infection

## Symptoms and conventional treatment

Dull to severe ache is felt that lasts for several hours. The most conventional method of treatment is taking recourse to pain killers but the side effects are wide and varied (see page 145).

## Yogic Treatment

When yoga is used as a method of treatment each type of body ache is treated differently.

**For uric acid:** Follow the yogic regime of inflammatory arthritis

**To throw the infections out:** Shankhapraksyalan is most effective. Also, take 1 gram of turmeric on an empty stomach every morning and evening

**For osteoporosis:** See the relevant section

**Growing pain:** Growing pain is a recurring phenomenon which occurs due to unbalanced hormonal secretions. The following yogic techniques should be practised to normalize glandular functions:

**To increase the healing energy**—surya namaskara

**To stabilize the glandular functions**—sarvangasana, chakrasana and ardhamatsyendrasana

**To improve the skeletal strength**—tadasana

**To rectify any structural defects**—ushtrasana

**To clear the energy channels**—nadisodhan pranayama

**To balance and soothe the nervous system**—bhramari pranayama

**To remove stress**—meditation and yoganidra to be practised in accordance with the age of the child

**To remove toxins**—laghoo shankhaprakshyalan once a week for two months and then once a month (recommended only for children above 15 years of age)

**For overworked body**—as well for growing pain, a massage with warm mustard oil mixed with a little camphor gives excellent result.

It is also important to maintain a well balanced diet in order to rectify any nutritional deficiencies.

........................................................................

# FROZEN SHOULDER

## What

Frozen shoulder generally results from stiffness of the shoulder ligaments.

## Why

- Overuse or misuse of the shoulder joints
- Lack of proper exercise

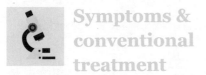 ## Symptoms & conventional treatment

It generally begins with pain and stiffness in the shoulder and an inability to lift the arm. There may

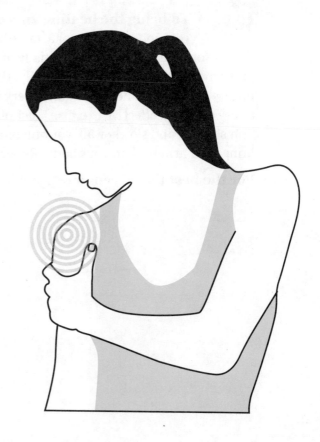

also be pain in the upper arm or neck. Patients tend not to move the affected arm which stiffens the ligaments causing it to break when strained. Anti-inflammatory drugs and pain killers are the most common methods of treatment. But the side effects can often be harmful (see page 145 for side effects).

## Yogic Treatment

- **To bring the healing energy to the shoulder**—Shoulder rotation—tadasana, hasta utthanasana, sarpasana and walking the fingers forward in adavasana. Initially, it may not be possible to do them properly. Do them anyhow. Gradually, they will become better. Walking the fingers on the wall should be done every now and then for speedy recovery. It is a very easy and effective exercise. Just place your hand on a wall, keeping the arm straight and slowly walk your fingers upward till the hurting point, then bring your arm back to your body. Repeat the exercise 5 to 10 times

- **For the best tissue repair**—yoganidra at bedtime

# GOUT

## What

Gout results from acidic fluid accumulation in a joint

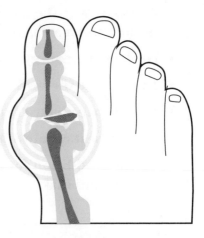

## Why

- Excessive intake of uric acid, far exceeding the body's capacity to eliminate it, which is then stored in the joints.

## Symptoms & conventional treatment

The symptoms occur with a sudden acute pain accompanied by swelling and redness in a single joint. Unless controlled, permanent joint damage and kidney problems can occur. Conventional treatment takes recourse to anti-inflammatory drugs, removal of the joint fluid syringe and uric acid lowering drugs. However the side effects can often lead to weakening of cartilage and the deterioration of joint tissues. For more on anti-inflammatory drugs (see page 146).

## Yogic Treatment

Yoga has proven beneficial in the treatment of gout

- **For better lymphatic drainage**—part 1 of pawanmuktasana

- **To rectify defects in the energy body**—chakki chalana, nauka sanchalana, tadasana

- **To increase the liver's capacity to detoxify**—dhanurasana, paschimottanasana

- **To wash away the acids**—laghoo shankha prakshyalana , 1 week with salt and for 2 to 3 months without it

- **To clear the energy pathways**—nadisodhana pranayama

- **To energize the brain**—kapalbhati pranayama

- **To improve chakra functions**—all chakra meditation

- **For the best repair of tissues**—yoganidra at bedtime

- **Optional addition for faster healing**—single chakra meditation on swadhisthana chakra

## Role of food

- **Cherry**—250 grams of cherry should be taken daily to lower uric acid level

- **Apples**—to neutralize the acid

- **Carrots**—to dissolve and prevent uric acid formation

Certain foods like cashew nuts and bajra (pearl millet) should be avoided as they have high uric acid. Protein intake should be substantially reduced as the end product of all protein is uric acid. If non-vegetarian food is a must, then take a small quantity of fish. However purine rich food such as sardine, red meat and alcohol must be avoided at all cost.

*Yoga and Diet for Ailments*

# HEADACHE (eye strain related)

## What

Overuse of the eyes and not resting them enough leads to headaches caused by eye strain as the muscles that contract to focus do not get a chance to relax fully

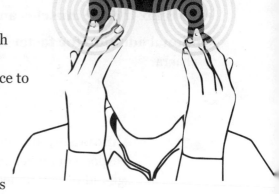

## Why

- Eyesight defect is a major cause for headaches

## Symptoms & conventional treatment

It often starts with a heaviness in the forehead that feels nice when pressed. Pain killers are generally used to provide relief but side effects are wide and many (see page 145).

## Yogic Treatment

If the eyesight is not affected, blinking frequently and relaxing the eyes can do wonders. But if the eyes are already weak, yoga can arrest and even reverse the deterioration. Try the following regime for 2 weeks before seeking medical treatment.

- **To strengthen the eye muscles**—eye exercises, sambhavi mudra, and tratak

- **To bring more blood to the eyes**—sarvangasana

- **To bring more healing energy to the eyes**—shanmukhi mudra

- **To de-stress**—mantra meditation

- **To relax the eye muscles and nerves**—palming, neti and yoganidra

**Optional addition for faster healing**—single chakra meditation on agnya chakra

### Role of food

- **Almonds**—7 almonds soaked overnight and ground with half a teaspoon of fennel and taken in the morning for 3 weeks is an age-old Indian remedy to improve eyesight

- **Cod liver oil, carrot, papaya, leafy vegetables**—these are rich in Vitamin A which helps in strengthening and restoring eyesight

# HEADACHE (migraine related)

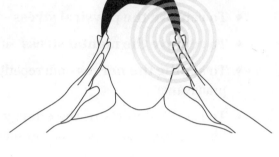

## What

Migraine is extreme discomfort in the head

## Why

- Stress, as it tenses up all the body tissues including that of the head

- Deficiencies of niacin, iron and potassium

- Disturbed glandular functions

## Symptoms & conventional treatment

Migraine starts with an intense throbbing pain, generally on one side of the head often accompanied by visions of sparkling lights or black spots. In some cases migraine may also lead to nausea and vomiting. Painkillers, cardiac drugs, anti-depressant, anti-seizure, anti-histamine and botox toxin are conventionally used to arrest the onset and for treatment of migraine, but these drugs are highly toxic, which is the reason some of them are contra-indicated during pregnancy and if there is kidney ailment, liver problem or high blood pressure. The symptoms are nausea, fever, changes in blood pressure, agitation, restlessness, hallucination seizure, and many more (see page 145 for the side effects of painkillers).

## Yogic Treatment

Kunjal is the most effective kriya for this problem. It has to be done every morning for 6 weeks and then twice a week for 6 months.

- **To remove the physical stress**—part 1 of pawanamuktasana

- **To remove the mental stress**—internal mantra repetition

- **To soothe the nerves**—om repetition for 10 minutes and bhramari pranayama

- **To rectify defects in the energy body**—tadasana, paschimottanasana, bhujangasana, shalbhasana and sheetli pranayama

- **To increase the healing energy**—suryanamaskar

- **To strengthen the nerves**—trikonasana

- **To bring more blood to the head**—sarvangasana, shashankasana

- **To improve glandular function**—sarvangasana, kandhrasana

- **To clear the energy pathways**—nadisodhan pranayama

- **For the best repair of tissues**—yoganidra at bedtime

- **Optional addition for faster healing**—single chakra meditation on agnya chakra

- **Mantra repetition**—om with blue mantra mala

# HEADACHE (tension related)

## What

Often headache can also arise due to tension of day-to-day life

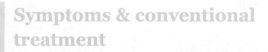

## Why

- Excessive mental work or extreme worry and anger can tense the muscles of the head and cause discomfort

## Symptoms & conventional treatment

This kind of headache generally arises from a dull pressing pain at the top, temples or back of the neck. Painkillers are preferred method of treatment as they provide quick but temporary relief and often the side effects are harmful. (see page 145)

## Yogic Treatment

- **To release the physical tension**—naukasana, part 1 of pawanamuktasana

- **To bring more blood to the head**—pada hastasana, sarvangasana
- **To relax the taut nerves**—bhramari pranayama, naukasana, sheetli pranayama
- **To bring more healing energy to the head**—sambhavi mudra
- **To de-stress**—breath awareness meditation
- **To relax deep**—short yoganidra, twice daily
- **Optional addition for faster healing**—single chakra meditation on agnya chakra

Just lying down in shavasana and counting the breaths backward from 100 to 1 relaxes the nerves and muscles, and gives immediate relief. However with continuous tension, if one has already developed high blood pressure then these methods may not help much. One needs to first normalize the pressure, which can be achieved in barely 3-4 days with a correct yogic regime. (Refer to *'Yoga for a Healthy Heart'* by the same author.)

3

# Digestive Disorders

Digestive problems such as acidity, gas and constipation can be extremely irritating, inconvenient and stressful. It can also lead to serious life threatening diseases including cancer, because improperly digested food remains unused in the cells and putrefies, making the body acidic and toxic. The kidneys and the liver get strained trying to eliminate these harmful substances. With continuous extra work they also become weak and ineffective and more toxins pile up making the body an ideal target for illness. What is worse is that curing these ailments can become difficult as the food that could have cured them now cannot be digested. Therefore, keeping the digestive system in top condition should be a priority.

# ACIDITY

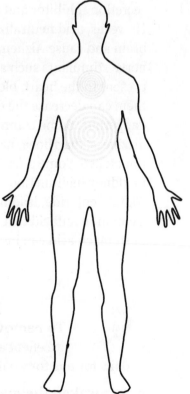

## What

Acidity can result from excessive and untimely acid secretion in the stomach

## Why

- Eating too much as it requires more acid for digestion
- Eating too fast. It leaves food in chunks which takes longer to be processed drawing more acid
- Regular consumption of rich acidic food
- Anxiety, especially during meals lead to acid secretion
- Inadequate intake of water leading to concentrated acid that is more eroding
- Acid producing foods and drinks
- Irregular meals
- Frequent eating as it means constant stimulation of acid producing organs
- Nutritional deficiencies, especially of Vitamin A, pantothenic acid, and sulfur

 ## Symptoms & conventional treatment

The more common symptoms of acidity are heartburn, acid reflux and lack of appetite. If neglected it can lead to any disease from ulcer to cancer. Acid secretion inhibitor and acid neutralizer are the most common forms of treatment. However, acid neutralizers contain aluminum which can get deposited in the brain and cause Alzheimer's. Acid secretion inhibitor works by suppressing the nerve stimulants such as histamine and H-receptors. As these chemicals are present in the heart, blood-vessels, bone marrow and pituitary, etc., suppressing them can decrease the efficiency of these important body parts which can be dangerous. Some common symptoms of reduced functions are headache, dizziness, diarrhoea, nausea, rashes, itching, constipation, swollen ankles and impotence. Some antacids lead to calcium deposits in the body which can result in kidney malfunction while some others react with the stomach acid and form sodium chloride, leading to sodium retention and edema. Sodium bicarbonate is a common antacid that destroys vitamins in the body. Lastly, persistent reduction of stomach acid can increase the body's susceptibility to intestinal pathogens.

## Yogic Treatment

- **To remove the extra acids from the stomach**—Kunjal is excellent and gives immediate relief. For the cure, it should be done daily for one to two months and followed by thrice a week for 2 to 3 months

- **To awaken the manipura chakra, the controller of the digestive system**—yogamudra asana, uddiyana bandha

- **To strengthen the digestive system**—part 2 of Pawanmuktasana

- **To increase the body's healing energy**—suryanamaskara

- **To clear the energy pathways**—nadisodhana pranayama

- **To improve liver function**—bhujangasana, shalabhasana and paschimottanasana

- **To calm the mind**—chanting om, bhramari pranayama, and internal mantra repetition
- **For the best repair of cells**—yoganidra at bedtime
- **Optional addition for faster healing**—single chakra meditation on manipura chakra

## Role of food

- **Cider vinegar**—a mixture of 1 tablespoon cider vinegar and the same quantity of honey with half a cup of hot water half an hour before meals is a common and effective remedy
- **Neem leaves (margosa)**—chewing 2 to 3 of these leaves helps in countering acidity
- **Isabgol**—soaked overnight in a glass of water and sipped in the morning on an empty stomach at least an hour before breakfast covers and protects the intestinal walls from the corroding acid, giving it a chance to heal
- **Banana and milk**—a mixture of these two together should be taken twice to thrice daily. Milk neutralizes the acid while banana has serotonin, a substance that controls acid secretion
- **Juices of ash gourd and bottle gourd**—to neutralize the existing acids
- **Gulkand (rose confection)**—after meals is an effective ayurvedic remedy
- **Basil leaves**—20 leaves with 1 tsp of honey taken for 2 to 3 months heals the affected tissues
- **Cloves, aniseed, and cardamom**—a combination of 2 cloves, few aniseed

and 1 cardamom after meals aid digestion. Cardamom also prevents putrefaction of food

- **Carrot and apple**—juice extracted from carrot and apple contain important digestive enzymes
- **Pomegranate, bel leaves (wood apple)**—tone up the liver
- **Saffron**—soothes the intestinal tract
- **Molasses**—highly alkaline in nature that neutralizes stomach acid

Simple, easy to digest food should be taken during the treatment period. Acid-forming food should be strictly avoided (see page 263).

Ayurveda further recommends avoidance of hot food and drinks.

## CONSTIPATION

### What

Inability to expel intestinal waste adequately can lead to constipation

### Why

- Lack of fibre in food
- Inadequate intake of water
- Excessive protein consumption
- Oily and fried food
- Obstruction in the intestine
- Hypothyroidism

- Deficiency of Vitamin B-complex
- Damaged intestine due to long term abuse
- Certain medicines, especially for high blood pressure, heart ailments, colon cancer and Parkinson's disease

## Symptoms & conventional treatment

The common symptoms are hard stool, bloating and not having the urge to pass stool regularly.

Laxatives are commonly used to treat constipation but they stimulate the enteric nerves. Too much stimulation can lead to their exhaustion. These nerves become weak leading to a sluggish intestine which can no longer function without medication. With external help, the intestine also becomes lazy and does not make an effort to improve its work. Secondly, laxatives cause excessive excretion of water, sodium and potassium which weakens the body muscles and makes them flabby. Lastly, laxatives of all kinds including the natural ones can flush out essential vitamins and minerals before they are absorbed.

## Yogic Treatment

- **To remove the accumulated toxic waste**—laghoo shankha prakshyalan—5 consecutive days with salt and then once a week for two three months where salt should be put in alternate weeks
- **To increase peristalsis or the intestinal movement**—matsya kridasana
- **To stretch and stimulate the intestine**—ushtrasana
- **To stretch and flex the intestine**—pada hastasana
- **To strengthen liver function and improve peristalsis**—paschimottanasana, merudandasana and tolangulasana

- **To exercise and strengthen the intestine**—part 2 of pawanmuktasana and abdominal breathing
- **To increase the internal heat for better digestion**—bhastrika pranayama
- **To increase the healing energy**—suryanamaskara
- **To clear the energy channels**—nadisodhana pranayama
- **To activate the mooladhara chakra that controls the elimination**—moola bandha
- **To de-stress and improve chakra function**—all chakra meditation
- **For better tissue rejuvenation**—yoganidra to sleep at night
- **Optional addition for faster healing**—single chakra meditation on mooladhara chakra

 ## Role of food

- **Harad powder**—take ½ teaspoon with warm water at bedtime. It is the most effective natural laxative
- **Trifala powder**—take ½ teaspoon after every meal to improve digestion
- **Isabgol**—take 1 teaspoon with 1 cup of warm milk in the evening to provide bulk to the intestinal content

A diet which includes fibre, and natural laxative foods such as green papaya, fig, date, apple, tamarind, millet, flax seeds, molasses, cod liver oil, barley and beet should be followed. Foods that induce constipation such as meat, cheese, egg, green banana, fried food, white flour, sugar and cold food and drinks should be avoided or taken in moderation. Protein intake should be further decreased. Sufficient water should be taken. Ayurveda recommends that water should be drunk warm.

*Yoga and Diet for Ailments*

# FOOD POISONING AND DIARRHOEA

## What

An upset stomach

## Why

- Infection
- Quantity of food exceeding body's capacity to digest
- Nutritional deficiencies, especially of Vitamin B-complex

## Symptoms & conventional treatment

The most common symptoms are stomach cramps, nausea, vomiting, frequent loose motion and fever. If left untreated it can lead to dehydration which in turn can result in brain damage. A course of antibiotics is generally used to treat the condition. But the side effects can lead to appetite loss and kills healthy bacteria in the intestine which are essential for digestion.

## Yogic Treatment

- Laghoo shankha prakshyalan should be done without delay to throw the infection out. It stops the diarrhoea almost instantaneously
- **To let the body heal completely**—yoganidra twice in the day

**Role of food**

- A diet of curd and rice, with water, should be taken. All other kinds of food should be avoided for a day or two

......................................................................

# GASTRITIS (chronic)

## What

Gastritis refers to the inflammation of the digestive tract

## Why

- Chronic acidity

- Insufficient digestive juices due to long-time abuse of the digestive system

- Nutritional deficiencies, especially of Vitamin A, pantothenic acid, and inositol

## Symptoms & conventional treatment

The symptoms are bloated stomach, abdominal discomfort, belching and burping, unclear motion.

and lack of appetite. If neglected the intestine becomes more and more inflamed and ultimately cannot move well. Waste and acids pile up, inviting hosts of diseases including some very serious ones. Antacid, intestine stimulator, digestive enzymes are used to provide relief but the side effects are wide and varied. Side effects from antacid have been covered under the section on Acidity and Constipation while the common side effects of enzymes are pain, bloating, burning, and diarrhoea. Taking enzymes discourages the digestive system to try and secrete their own. It can lead to the atrophy of the gland. Some enzymes destruct the natural existence of lipases upsetting fat digestion and damaging the large intestine. This in turn ups the risk of fibroid and colonopathy.

## Yogic Treatment

In addition to the yogic regime for acidity, the following practises should be followed:

- **To increase peristalsis**—matsya kridasana
- **To bring back the balance in humour production**—bhastrika pranayama
- **To reduce the humour 'vata', i.e., gas**—suryabheda pranayama
- **To stimulate the secretion of pancreatic enzymes**—ardha matsyendrasana and gomukhasana
- **To improve the liver function**—tolangulasana, paschimottanasana, bhujangasana
- **To eliminate the gas-producing bacteria**—guru shankha prakshyalana is the most effective. Fasting with urine is the next best. Taking urine in any case kills all germs. If none of these are possible, then laghoo shankha prakshyalana, along with the right food and natural medicine will help
- **Optional addition for faster healing**—single chakra meditation on manipura chakra

## Role of food

If there is acidity, the diet pattern for that ailment has to be followed:

- **Amaltas**—is extremely beneficial. Take an amla sized ball of the paste of the leaves with ½ cup of warm water in the morning on empty stomach

- **Harad, black pepper, black salt, rock salt**—mix the powder of harad, black pepper, black salt and rock salt and have ½ teaspoon of it after meals or whenever your stomach feels heavy

- **Cloves**—Push cloves into an apple and keep it covered in a bowl for 21 days. Remove the cloves and store in a bottle. Chew 2 of them after every meal

- **Ginger, fennel, coriander, cumin, carrot, and black rock salt**—to increase gastric juices

- **Nutmeg, thyme, peppermint, and alfalfa**—to promote appetite

- **Papaya**—contains digestive enzymes

- **Barley sprout, oats, saffron, and aloe vera**—to soothe the inflamed lining

- **Fresh curd, dates**—to repair the damaged flora

- **Bel (wood apple) and pro-biotic**—to kill the harmful intestinal bacteria

- **Asafetida (in curries)**—to reduce gas

Fresh curd (should not be sour) diluted with a glass of water and mixed with salt and roasted cumin powder is excellent. It is important to avoid gas-forming food such as leafy vegetables, beans, cheese, milk and all root vegetables except carrot, high fibre vegetables, legumes (except green gram), cauliflower, brinjal and non-vegetarian food (except light fish and a small quantity of chicken), as well as mustard, and watermelon. Also acid forming food should be avoided (see page 263). Ayurveda further recommends to drink ½ cup of very hot water after meals for 3 months, and to avoid cold drinks and cold food during that period. It is also advised to take a nap of half an hour in the afternoon after lunch and walk 100 steps after meals.

*Yoga and Diet for Ailments*

# PILES

## What

Piles results from swollen blood vessels at the rectum

## Why

- Chronic constipation that involves straining to pass stool

## Symptoms & conventional treatment

The symptoms are bleeding and tenderness during passing stool. If left untreated, it can lead to rectum cancer. Anesthetic application and surgery are the conventional forms of treatment. However anesthetic creams thin and damage the skin while surgery is not always effective and the problem almost always returns.

## Yogic Treatment

The yogic regime for constipation should be followed in addition to the following:

- **To bring prana to the affected part**—ashwini mudra
- **To drain the stagnant blood**—sarvangasana. The benefits are still more if both the practises are combined
- **Optional addition for faster healing**—single chakra meditation on mooladhara chakra

**Role of food:**

- **Apricots, figs and honey**—regular use of apricot helps to cure it, so do figs, and honey
- **Banana**—ripe (but not overtly) with cardamom at bedtime
- **Curry leaves**—tender curry leaves with honey
- **Radish, beet**—juice extracted from radish and beet leaves

. . . . . . . . . . . . . . . . . . . . . . . . . . . . . . . . . . . . . . . . . . . . . . . . . . . . . . . . . . . . . . . . . . . . . . . .

# SWALLOWING DIFFICULTY

## What

Although not a commonly heard-of ailment, many people suffer from difficulty in swallowing food

## Why

- Ulcer in the food pipe due to frequent acid reflux
- Malfunctioning of the muscles of the throat or esophagus
- Nutritional deficiencies especially of iron, and Vitamin B-complex

## Symptoms and conventional treatment

The symptoms are inability to swallow, discomfort in the chest during the passage of food and regurgitation of food. When left untreated it can lead to cancer of the esophagus and there is a risk of food getting into the wind pipe. Muscle relaxant and antacids are used to provide relief. However prolonged use of muscles relaxant weakens all the muscles in the body. For side effects of antacid please refer to section on Acidity.

## Yogic Treatment

In addition to the yogic regime for acidity the following practises should be done

- **To exercise the throat area**—simhasana

- **To bring more blood to the throat**—sarvangasana and pada hastasana

- **To draw the healing energy to the throat**—ujjayi pranayama and shanmukhi mudra

- **To strengthen the entire nervous system**—trikonasana

- **Optional addition for faster healing**—single chakra meditation on manipura chakra

## Role of food

- **Yeast, amla (Indian gooseberry) and honey**—provide relief

Also a well-balanced diet with some extra iron rich and alkaline food such as raisins, jaggery, molasses must be followed

••••••••••••••••••••••••••••••••••••••••••••••••••••••••••••••••

# ULCER

## What

Ulcers are open wounds in the stomach or duodenum

## Why

- High acidity
- Nutritional deficiencies especially of Vitamin A and pantothenic acid

 ## Symptoms & conventional treatment

Symptoms are burning in the stomach, that is relieved by drinking milk, stomach ache, nausea and vomiting, tenderness in the affected area, lack of appetite and bloating after meals. Often there is a gnawing stomach pain that increases after taking food in the case of stomach ulcer and decreases in duodenum ulcer. If the wound becomes deep, it perforates the digestive tract, spilling the acidic content into the abdominal cavity with serious consequences. Sometimes the ulcer perforates a major blood-vessel which can be life threatening. Acid secretion suppressants and surgery are commonly used to treat this condition. But surgery cannot guarantee a cure if the acid secretion remains the same while the suppressants suppress the nerve stimulators, turning the entire system sluggish.

## Yogic Treatment

The following practises should be followed in the beginning till the ulcer heals and the pain is gone

- **To mobilize the healing energy**—part 1 of pawanmuktasana with prana awareness
- **To draw more blood to the stomach for healing**—vajrasana whenever possible
- **To soothe the nerves**—bhramari pranayama and chanting om
- **To clear the energy pathways**—nadisodhan pranayama

- **To slow down the hyperactive digestive system**—sheetli pranayama

- **To remove stress**—internal mantra repetition

- **To relax and rejuvenate**—yoganidra at bedtime and sometime during the day

- **To normalize chakra function**—repetition of the mantra 'Ram'

After the initial healing, add the following:

- **To improve liver function**—pascimottanasana, tolangulasana. dhanurasana

- **To improve pancreatic function**—ardha matsyendrasana

- **Optional addition for faster healing**—single chakra meditation on manipura chakra

## Role of food

- **Banana**—fully ripe mashed banana with milk. Banana contains serotonin that prevents acid secretion; milk neutralizes the acid while Vitamin C of banana helps in healing

- **Mushroom, pumpkin seeds and wheat germ**—contain zinc which speeds up healing

In the beginning, juices extracted from cabbage mixed with grape juice, apple juice and carrot juice should be taken along with soft boiled rice, banana and honey. Later other non-acidic food such as porridge of ground wheat, barley or semolina, and non-sour fruits can be added to the diet. Normal food should be introduced one at a time to know if any of them is unsuitable. Small meals should be taken frequently, so as not to leave the stomach empty for the acid to come in direct contact with the sore. Acidic food should be avoided for at least a year (see page 263).

# ULCERATIVE COLITIS

## What

Ulcerative colitis are wounds and inflammation in the colon.

## Why

- Chronic acidity
- Infection
- Stress, as it leads to acid secretion

## Symptoms & conventional treatment

Symptoms are loose motion, abdominal pain, joint pain, blood in stool, skin lesions, weight loss and urgent bowel movement. If allowed to become chronic, it turns cancerous. Also, nutrients are not absorbed due to the unhealthy condition of the intestine, leading to various other health problems. Anti-inflammatory drug, anti-biotic, peristalsis inhibitor, corticosteroid and surgery are often taken recourse to remove a part of or the entire colon. Side effects are often harmful.

## Yogic Treatment

In the beginning the following should be practised:

- **To de-stress**—internal mantra repetition, chanting om and its mental repetition

- **To relax**—Yoganidra (twice daily) and counting the breaths backward from 100 to 1 in shavasana (2 to 3 times daily)

- **To mobilize the healing energy**—part 1 of pawanmuktasana

- **To soothe the stressed stomach nerves**—ananda madirasana, bhramari pranayama , sheetli pranayama, shitkari pranayama

- **To bring more blood to the digestive system for healing**—vajrasana. It should be done after meals and whenever possible

- **To clear the energy pathways**—nadisodhan pranayama

- **When condition improves add**—bhujangasana, ardha shalabhasana, paschimottanasana and shashankasana

- **When strength returns** do all the asanas for acidity and sarvangasana

- **Optional addition for faster healing**—single chakra meditation on manipura chakra

## Role of food

- **Amaltas leaves**—an amla sized ball of the paste should be taken with ½ cup of warm water in the morning on empty stomach to repair the intestine

- **Bel (wood apple)**—to tone up the intestine

A diet of milk and rice porridge (should be very soft), milk with mashed banana, green coconut water, and wheatgrass juice should be taken in the beginning. They are easy to digest and provide all the necessary nutrients. Molasses and honey give very good results as well. Sour, salty, sweet and spicy food should be avoided.

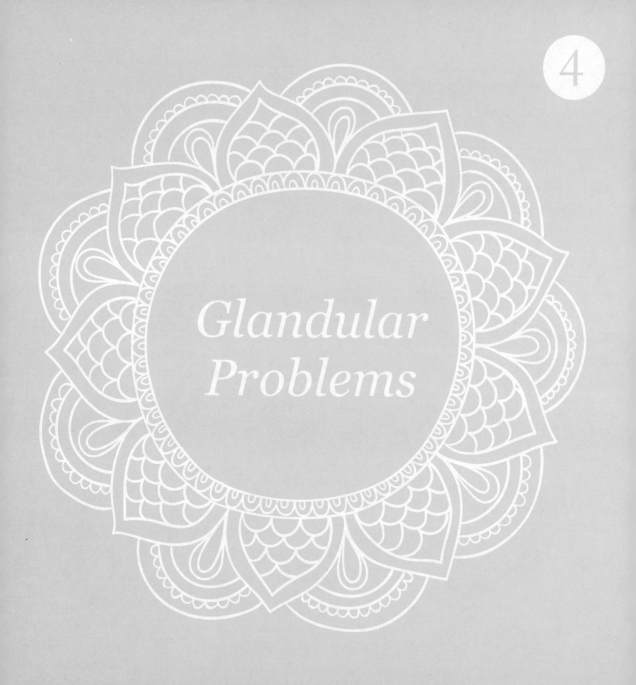

4

*Glandular Problems*

All our bodily functions
are regulated by
hormones which are
secreted by glands.
When these body parts
malfunction, the
required amount of
chemicals are not
produced, and the
system goes haywire
resulting in various
diseases.

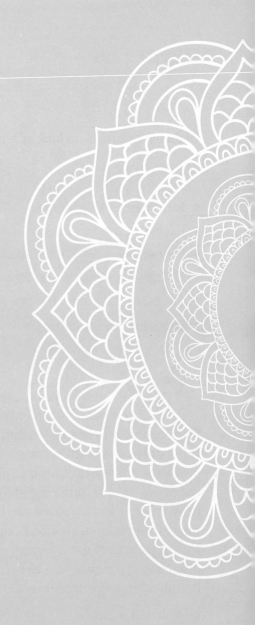

# DIABETES

## What

Diabetes results from lack of hormone insulin

## Why

- Inherited weak pancreas
- Excessive intake of sugar, leading to pancreatic exhaustion
- Sedentary life where the sugar in the blood is not used up
- Nutritional deficiencies, especially of chromium
- Stress, as it disturbs the smooth functioning of the system
- Excessive toxins in the body

## Symptoms & conventional treatment

The most common symptoms are frequent urination, increased volume of urine, increased appetite, weight loss, excessive thirst, fatigue, blurred vision, skin and bladder infection and delayed healing of wound. If left untreated it affects every tissue in the body adversely leading to serious problems of the heart, brain, kidneys, liver, skin, and nerves. Left uncontrolled, the disease can be fatal. Hypoglycemic drugs, insulin administration are most conventional and favoured methods of treatment. However the side effects can range from itching, skin rash, upset stomach, constipation, gas, bloating, anemia, weight gain, liver diseases and kidney malfunction. Also, supplying insulin discourages the pancreas to make an effort to secrete the hormone. The gland becomes lazy, affecting its other functions adversely.

## Yogic treatment

- **To revive the pancreas**—guru shankh prakshyalan is extremely effective. If that is not possible, do laghoo shankha prakshyalan for 40 days as it yields almost the same result.

- **To bring more blood to the pancreas**—ardha matsyendrasana, dhanurasana, supta vajrsana and yogamudrasana

- **To send prana to this gland**—gomukhasana

- **To increase the body's healing energy**—surya namaskara

- **To relax the nerves**—bhramari pranayama

- **To clear the energy pathways**—nadisodhan pranayama

- **To de-stress**—internal mantra repetition

- **To speed up healing**—yoganidra, preferably with the therapeutic mantra

- **Optional addition for faster healing**—single chakra meditation on manipura chakra

## Role of food

- **Bitter gourd**—½ glass of bitter gourd juice with equal amount of water in the morning on empty stomach helps stimulate the pancreas. In the initial stage, the reversal can be dramatic

- **Fenugreek powder**—½ teaspoon after meals

- **Curry leaves, jamun (Indian blue berry), and amla powder (Indian gooseberry)**—are equally effective in stimulating the pancreas

- **Mushroom, pumpkin seeds, and wheat germ**—as they contain zinc which increases the effectiveness of insulin

- **Ragi**—is a beneficial cereal, as it is digested slowly, i.e. with the starch is released slowly
- **Coconut jelly**—as it has no fat or starch
- **Guar (cluster beans)**—it checks quick absorption of carbohydrates
- **Yeast**—has high amount of chromium. It also has high glucose tolerance factor

It is important to follow a strict diet and restrict calories by adding more fibrous food such as oats, leafy vegetables and carrots

# ENLARGED LIVER

## What

The size of the liver increases

## Why

- Obesity
- Chronic alcoholism
- Prolonged use of steroid
- Water retention
- Excessive toxins
- Pathogens

## Symptoms

Enlarged liver is accompanied by pain and tenderness in the right abdomen. As the liver removes toxins from the blood, when it cannot do that effectively, the body is slowly poisoned leading to many serious ailments. Often the causative factor is treated while the source of the problem is left ignored.

## Yogic treatment

The workload on the liver must be reduced by first removing the toxins from the system and by taking suitable food

- **To remove toxins**—laghoo shankha prakshyalana—for 5 days, then once a week for 2-3 months. Salt should be used every alternate week

- **To bring more blood and healing energy to the gland**—paschimottanasana, bhujangasana, vajrasana, shashankasana, meru wakrasana

- **To rectify defects in the energy body**—merudandasana, tolangulasana, veerasana

- **To energize**—suryabheda pranayama

- **To clear the energy pathways**—nadisodhan pranayama

- **To activate the concerned chakra**—uddiyana bandha

- **To de-stress**—internal mantra repetition

- **For the best rejuvenation of tissues**—yoganidra at bedtime

- **Optional addition for faster healing**—single chakra meditation on manipura chakra

## Role of food

- **Green Papaya**—milk extracted from green papaya gives excellent result in 2 to 3 weeks. Around 20 drops on a piece of bread taken on an empty stomach are more than enough to provide satisfying results

- **Apple juice**—to cleanse the liver

- **Bel and long pepper**—around 3 leaves of bel (wood apple) and the powder of 1 long pepper help to tone up the liver

- **Alfalfa sprouts, carrot, celery, and basil**— improve appetite

- **Sugarcane juice, apricot, pomegranate juice, drumsticks, beet, and cooked fenugreek**—improve liver function

Further it is important to avoid fried foods and foods that are yellow in colour.

· · · · · · · · · · · · · · · · · · · · · · · · · · · · · · · · · · · · · · · · · · · · · · · · · · · · · ·

# ENLARGED PROSTATE

## What

Enlarged prostate refers to a swollen prostate gland.

## Why

- Degeneration due to aging

- Lack of correct exercise

 ## Symptoms & conventional treatment

The common symptoms are frequent urge to urinate, difficulty in starting urination and decreased force in the urine flow. If ignored the bladder can get infected and the kidney damaged. Muscle relaxant, hormone blocker and surgery are often the preferred methods of treatment. However the side effects are many. With relaxed muscles, one can lose complete control over urination. Hormones blockers suppress the nervous system, which is harmful for the nerve health. Also, with less male hormone, there may be loss of libido and enlarged breasts. Dizziness, nausea, headache, digestive system problems, sinus congestion, and eye disorder are some of the common effects of the medication. And surgery may lead to impotence.

## Yogic treatment

- **To mobilize the healing energy in the body**—part 1 of pawan muktasana series

- **To exercise and tone the gland**—vajroli

- **To draw more blood to the prostate**—merudandasana, naukasana

- **To draw more healing energy to the gland**—veerasana, moola bandha

- **To clear the energy pathways**—nadisodhan pranayama

- **To de-stress**—internal mantra repetition

- **For the best tissue rejuvenation**—yoganidra at bedtime

- **Optional addition for faster healing**—single chakra meditation on swadhisthana chakra

## Role of food

- **Musk melon seeds**—if taken daily, is likely to shrink the gland

*Yoga and Diet for Ailments*

# HYPOTHYROIDISM

## What

Hypothyroidism arises from lack of the thyroxin hormone

## Why

- Nutritional deficiencies, especially of iodine
- Stress, as it disturbs all bodily functions
- Heredity

## Symptoms & conventional treatment

The common symptoms are weight gain, lethargy, depression, fatigue, decreased heartbeat, intolerance to cold, slow function of the body and mind, constipation, dry skin and hair, abnormal menstrual problems, brittle nails, memory impairment, swollen face and feet, swollen neck, sometimes leading to goiter and ringing in the ears. If hypothyroidism is left untreated it hampers physical and mental growth in children. In extreme cases, it can cause dwarfism, mental retardation and heart failure. Ingestion of thyroid hormone is the preferred method of treatment. However with hormone supplement, the gland can atrophy, affecting its other functions. Prolonged use of large doses can lead to osteoporosis and left ventricular hypertrophy. The common side effects are fatigue, headache, insomnia, anxiety and excessive sweating

## Yogic treatment

- **To increase body's healing energy**—suryanamaskara
- **To bring more blood to the thyroid**—padahastasana, sarvangasana
- **To stretch and massage the gland**—supta vajrasana
- **To bring more prana to this gland**—vipareet karani mudra, jalandhara bandha and ujjayi pranayama
- **To improve the entire glandular system**—kandhrasana
- **To stimulate pituitary, the master gland**—pranamasana. If this asana is not possible then do shashankasana
- **To clear the energy pathways**—nadi sodhana pranayama
- **To relax the nerves**—bhramari pranayama
- **To de-stress**—internal mantra repetition
- **To speed up healing**—therapeutic yoganidra
- **Optional addition for faster healing**—single chakra meditation on vishuddhi chakra

## Role of food

- **Sea weeds, sea fish and onions**—they have iodine, the constituent of thyroxin
- **Whole grain, nuts and leafy vegetables**—they contain the mineral manganese which is essential for forming thyroxin in the body
- **Coconut**—it improves thyroid health

A diet rich in beans, carrots, lettuce, peach, spinach, broccoli, cabbage, brussels sprouts and soya products must be avoided as they inhibit thyroxin production.

# POLYCYSTIC OVARY

## What

Polycystic ovary refers to multiple growths on the ovaries

## Why

- Stress leading to disturbed glandular functions
- Nutritional deficiencies
- Acidic system

## Symptoms & conventional treatment

Unpredictable menstrual cycles, absence of periods and extreme pain during periods are some of the common symptoms. If left untreated it can lead to infertility and excessive facial hair. Hormone supplements and diuretic are commonly used to treat this disorder. However, supplements can make the gland atrophy while diuretic removes salt from the body, which can disturb the electrolyte balance of the system. That in turn can lead to muscle cramps and even heart attack. As these drugs manipulate the nerves, some common problems that develop are nausea, fatigue, drowsiness, headache, diarrhoea, cramps, rashes, and hair loss. It can also mean an increased risk of ovarian tumor.

## Yogic treatment

- **To exercise the ovaries**—chakki chalana, nauka sanchalana, leg lock

- **To draw more healing energy to the ovaries**—marjari asana, shashankasana, veerasana

- **To draw more blood to the pituitary, the controlling gland**—sarvangasana

- **To increase the healing energy in the body**—suryanamaskara

- **For better glandular health**—chakrasana, kandhrasana

- **To clear the energy pathways**—nadisodhan pranayama

- **To relax the nerves**—bhramari pranayama

- **To burn toxins**—bhastrika pranayama

- **To de-stress**—mind vision meditation

- **For better tissue rejuvenation**—yoganidra at bedtime

- **Optional addition for faster healing**—single chakra meditation on swadhishthana chakra

It is further important to follow a non acidic and balanced diet to treat this condition.

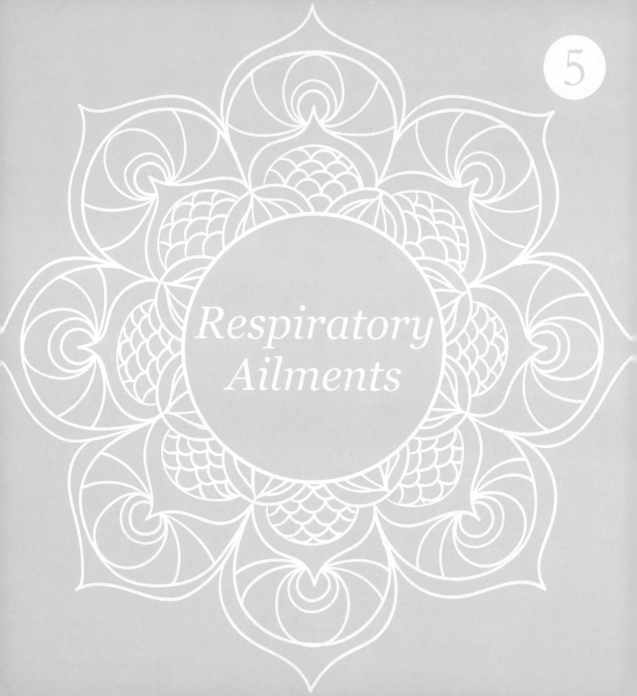

5

*Respiratory Ailments*

The 60 trillion cells that constitute the human body need a continuous supply of oxygen to survive and function properly. This has to be ensured by taking an adequate amount of air into the lungs. But if the respiratory tract becomes inflamed (due to the problems mentioned in the following pages), the intake of air is greatly reduced and the entire system is deprived of this valuable life-giving substance. This can have a detrimental effect on one's general health and well-being. Yoga can effectively and quickly alleviate most of these respiratory problems.

# ASTHMA

Constriction of the airways, leading to breathing difficulty

- Heredity
- Stress, as it disturbs all bodily functions
- Allergens that irritate the mucus membrane and cause swelling
- Nutritional deficiencies, especially that of Vitamins A and D

## Symptoms & conventional treatment

Wheezing, tightness in the chest, laboured breathing and an increased pulse rate are some of the symptoms of asthma. It can lead to poor health and growth. A severe asthma attack can be very distressing, and in extreme cases, it can also be fatal.

Conventional treatments may include use of bronco dilators, oxygen therapy and steroids. However, bronco dilator has poor cardiac action. This can lead to high blood pressure, and when blood pressure lowering medicines are taken to control it, the severity of an asthmatic attack can increase.

Similarly, steroids can damage the brain cells and oxygen therapy makes the body intolerant to carbon dioxide. In higher altitudes, and even with a little exertion, an asthmatic patient may show signs of distress.

**To avert an attack**—yoganidra should be practised at the first sign of an attack to stop it immediately. Prior to the actual attack, if there is a cold or a cough, laghoo shankha prakshyalana or even kunjal can be of great help. To cure the ailment completely, practising the following yogic asanas is necessary:

- **To increase the healing energy**—suryanamaskara

- **To open up the lungs**—marjariasana, hasta utthanasana and chin mudra

- **To bring more blood to the lungs for healing**—shashankasana

- **To promote the secretion of cortisone**—ushtrasana, akarna dhanurasana

- **To clear the energy pathways**—nadisodhana pranayama

- **To increase body heat**—bhastrika pranayama

- **To stimulate the chakra**—jalandhara bandh

- **To de-stress**—cathartic meditation

- **To relax for best tissue rejuvenation**—yoganidra at bedtime

- **To free the body cells clogged with mucus**—laghoo shankha prakshyalan for 4 to 5 days in the beginning and then twice to thrice a month for 6 months. Thereafter, you can practise it once a month or whenever the need arises

- **Optional addition for faster healing**—single chakra meditation on vishuddhi chakra

## Role of food

- **Basil leaves:** It has anti-mucus properties. Keep 7 basil leaves with water in a conch and leave it overnight, and take it in the morning.

However, due to the high level of mercury content in basil leaves, they should not be chewed, as it could damage the teeth. You should break the leaves into small pieces and swallow them. For children, it can be ground into a paste. Babies with asthmatic tendencies should be kept in the vicinity of basil plants.

Your diet should be light and easy to digest, so that you can save energy for the healing process. Heat-producing food like garlic, ginger, saffron, sesame, jaggery, turmeric and honey should be included in your daily diet. At the same time, avoid all kinds of mucus-forming foods like rice, banana, milk, curd, lady's finger and arbi (colocasia). Pulses like horse gram, black gram and kidney beans are hard to digest and can cause harm to the body. You should also stay away from cold foods and drinks.

· · · · · · · · · · · · · · · · · · · · · · · · · · · · · · · · · · · · · · · · · · · · · · · · · · · · · · · · · · · · · · · · · · · ·

# BRONCHITIS

## What

Inflammation of the mucus membrane of the respiratory tract

## Why

- Viral infection that generally spreads to the chest after common cold
- Smoking
- Dust
- Air pollution
- Nutritional deficiencies, especially that of Vitamins A and C

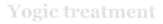

## Symptoms & conventional treatment

The most common symptoms of bronchitis are chest congestion and cough. If untreated, the disease becomes chronic, resulting in constant coughing and breathlessness. Moreover, continuous lack of oxygen can be detrimental to the overall health. In severe cases, it can also shorten lifespan drastically. Antibiotics, bronco dilator and oxygen therapy are the most common forms of treatment.

## Yogic treatment

- **To remove chest congestion**—laghoo shankha prakshyalan and kunjal. It should be practised daily till the chest feels free of congestion
- **To heal the wind pipes**—shashankasana, sarvangasana
- **To open up the lungs**—marjariasana, chin mudra
- **To strengthen the chest**—matsyasana, abdominal breathing
- **To activate the concerned chakra**—jalandhara bandha
- **To de-stress and speed up the healing process**—all chakra meditations
- **To relax, for the best tissue rejuvenation**—yoganidra at bedtime
- **Optional addition for faster healing**—single chakra meditation on vishuddhi chakra

## Role of food

- **Trikatu:** Take ½ teaspoon of long pepper, black pepper and dry ginger, and mix it with ½ teaspoon of triphala. Having this mixture twice every day generates body heat that helps in melting and expelling the mucus

- **Fenugreek and pepper:** An infusion of fenugreek and pepper, if taken every night, can have a dilatory effect on the bronchial pipes
- **Ginger and fenugreek:** The infusion acts as an expectorant

The diet to be followed should be the same as that of asthma

## COMMON COLD

### What

Infection of the nasal passage, mostly viral

### Why

- Exposure to cold
- Low immunity
- Stress, since it lowers immunity
- Nutritional deficiencies, especially that of potassium, silicon, and Vitamins A and C

### Symptoms & conventional treatment

The most common symptoms are runny nose, congestion in the nasal passage, watery eyes, sneezing, coughing, sore throat, heaviness in the head and fever.

Common cold is not a very serious problem because of the self-limiting nature of the cold virus. It dies after having run its course.

Antibiotics, anti-allergy drugs and Vitamin C tablets are the usual forms of treatment. But antibiotics, as the name suggests, work only on bacteria and have no effect on viruses.

## Yogic treatment

- **To remove the infection**—kunjal and neti can remove the infection quickly. Shanmukhi mudra too is very effective

- **To build up immunity post infection**—a well-rounded yogic regime for general fitness should be followed regularly. If possible, suryanamaskara should also be included in the regime. This practise is an excellent way to build immunity. People, especially children, who do not have any health problems can maintain good health by practising suryanamaskara every day
  (For yogic regimes, please see **Yoga for Busy People** by the same author).

## Role of food

- **Turmeric**: take ¼ teaspoon of turmeric in the morning 45 minutes after kunjal. Its anti-viral and anti-bacterial properties help kill the infection

- **Garlic**: Having garlic toast (see recipe on page 277) or garlic at any time of the day can work as an effective remedy because of its anti-viral and anti-bacterial properties

- **Kadha** (see recipe on page 277): Helps increase body heat and to dry up the mucus. You should have it 2 to 3 times every day

- **Pumpkin soup:** Helps expel mucus

People suffering from common cold should avoid having banana, curd, rice, cold food and drinks. Fasting for a day (or half a day) and consuming only green tea, kadha and water is the most effective natural treatment. Massaging the soles with mustard oil with spices (see page 279) is an excellent therapy, especially for children who cannot do the yogic treatment. Do it at bedtime for maximum benefit.

Garlic cloves can be strung as a necklace and put around a baby's neck for relief.

......................................................................

# COUGH

## What

The reflex to clear the respiratory tract

## Why

- Infection such as influenza and tuberculosis

- Inflamed vocal cord

- Smoking

- Allergies

- Asthma

- Nutritional deficiencies, especially of potassium, silicon and Vitamins A and C

 **Symptoms & conventional treatment**

Iirritation in the throat, breathlessness and stuffy nose are the most common symptoms. Since coughing contracts the air passage, if it happens frequently, the mucus membrane of the respiratory tract would remain inflamed, causing inadequate oxygen inflow into the lungs, affecting one's general health adversely.

Antibiotics, cough syrups with a combination of anti-histamines, expectorants, cough suppressants, and bronco dilators are the usual forms of treatment. Cough suppressants can depress the cough centre in the medulla, inhibiting the cough reflex. When done excessively, it can also permanently depress the nervous system.

## Yogic treatment

- **To remove the infection**—kunjal, shanmukhi mudra

  Build your resistance by following the yogic regime for general fitness

(See *Yoga for Busy People* by the same author).

## Role of food

- **Turmeric:** It is a potent killer of all kinds of infections. Mix ¼ teaspoon of turmeric in half a cup of hot water and sip it slowly. Have this water twice or thrice every day
- **Harad:** It helps produce internal heat that aids in the drying up of the mucus. Fry 3 to 4 pieces of this dry fruit in ghee (clarified butter) till it turns almost black. Then keep a piece of it in your mouth till it dissolves. Have this 3 to 4 times every day
- **Yogic tea with honey:** It helps soothe the throat (see page 278)
- **Basil and ginger:** A juice of these two ingredients acts as a natural expectorant

*Yoga and Diet for Ailments*

Your diet should be light and you should eat less so that the energy saved can be used for healing. Avoid cold and mucus-producing foods such as curd, banana and milk products. If you must have milk, add a pinch of turmeric to cut its cooling properties.

The above mentioned foods can heat up the stomach and may cause other health problems. To prevent that you can keep a wet towel on your navel for 20 to 30 minutes (the towel should be placed in such a way that it does not cover the ribcage). You can keep the neck warm by wrapping a woolen scarf around it.

••••••••••••••••••••••••••••••••••••••••••••••••••••••••••••••••••••••••••••

# SINUSITIS

## What

Inflammation of the lining of the sinus cavity

## Why

- Infection that spreads to the sinuses after a common cold
- Infection from a diseased dental root
- Deviated spectrum
- Nutritional deficiencies especially that of Vitamins A, C and D

## Symptoms & conventional treatment

Blocked nose, headache and heaviness in the head are the common symptoms. Some other symptoms can be headache, rapid heartbeat, fatigue, acne and trembling. If left untreated, there is a risk of the infection spreading to the facial bones or to the brain—both of which are dangerous conditions. There are instances when sinusitis has lead to paralysis. Antibiotics, nasal drops to de-congest, and surgery are the usual forms of treatment. Nasal drops are mostly steroids that reduce the inflammation and dry up the nasal lining. Using drops would make the nostrils extremely dry. It also increases the risk of sinus infection. Prolonged use of nasal drops can also dull the sense of smell.

## Yogic treatment

- **To de-congest the nose and remove the infection**—neti (starting with thrice a day, the number of repetitions can be reduced as the health improves) and shanmukhi mudra
- **To increase the healing energy**—surya namaskara
- **To increase the body heat**—bhastrika and kapalbhati pranayama
- **To strengthen the lungs**—abdominal breathing, ushtrasana, dwikonasana, and matsyasana
- **To de-stress while energizing the brain tissues**—mind vision meditation
- **To relax for the best tissue rejuvenation**—yoganidra at bedtime
- **Optional addition for faster healing**—single chakra meditation on vishuddhi chakra

## Role of food

The role of food is the same as in the case of asthma.

Whenever you feel your nose getting choked, apply a little warm spiced mustard oil (see page 279).

*Yoga and Diet for Ailments*

# TONSILITIS

## What

Inflammation of the outer covering of the wind pipe

## Why

- Viral infection
- Nutritional deficiencies of Vitamins A and C, as that leads to weak immunity

## Symptoms & conventional treatment

Sore throat, experiencing pain while swallowing food, fever and chills are some common symptoms. If it becomes chronic, the patient would be forced to breathe from the mouth which can adversely affect both his or her physical and mental abilities. Antibiotics and surgery are the most common forms of treatment. as tonsillitis is the body's first line of defense against invading pathogens, removing them by surgery makes the body vulnerable to serious, infectious diseases, while anti-biotic weaken the entire system. But if the infection is severe, it becomes necessary to take the medication without delay.

## Yogic treatment

- **To kill the infection** — Laghoo Shankha Prakshyalan
- **To heal the throat and prevent further infection—**
simhasana (This is most effective when done facing the morning sun; but do

not look at the sun directly as that can damage the retina) and shanmukhi mudra

- **To bring more blood to the throat**—shashankasana, sarvangasana and pada hastasana
- **To bring more prana to the throat**—ujjayi pranayama
- **To soothe the throat**—sheetli pranayama
- **To increase the healing energy**—suryanamaskara
- **To increase the inner heat**—bhastrika pranayama
- **To de-stress and to activate the chakras**—all chakra meditations
- **To relax and for the best tissue rejuvenation**—yoganidra at bedtime
- **Optional addition for faster healing**—single chakra meditation on vishuddhi chakra

 ### Role of food

Green tea with rock salt and lots of garlic can provide relief. Keep the throat covered and warm at all times

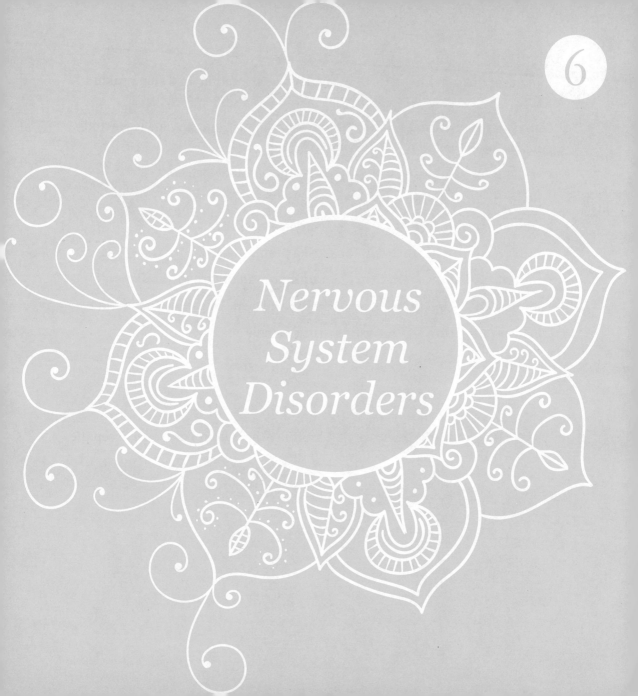

6

Nervous
System
Disorders

Brain—the apex of the nervous system—controls every little function of the body, be it the blinking of the eyes or the pounding of the heart. It receives data from every cell, analyses them, decides what is to be done and sends out the required instructions. The messages from the body parts to the brain, and from the brain to the body cells, are carried out by the nervous system. When this system becomes weak and diseased, the messages are not delivered as required. This affects all the bodily functions. Worse is, if the brain cells die, they do not regenerate. But yoga can strengthen the existing weakened nerves and arrest the degeneration.

Although I have covered only the ailments I have treated successfully, I am sure the following practises can help treat other nervous system ailments such as Alzheimer's disease, myasthenia gravis, etc.

# COMMON PRACTICES FOR ALL NERVOUS SYSTEM AILMENTS

- **To stretch and exercise the nerves**—part 1 of pawanmuktasana series
- **To strengthen the nervous system**—eka pada pranamasana, natavara, nataraja and trikonasana
- **To clear the energy pathways**—nadisodhan pranayama
- **To relax the nerves of the head**—neti
- **For the best tissue rejuvenation**—yoganidra at bedtime

# COMMON FOOD FOR THE NERVOUS SYSTEM

- **Apple, mango and soya:** Rich in glutamic acid (a substance which helps repair the nerves)
- **Spinach, peas, broccoli and asparagus:** These are rich in folic acid which is needed by glutamic acid for its function
- **Sprouts, legumes, meat, fish, egg, milk and milk products:** These are essential nerve foods rich in Vitamin B-complex
- **Fish and seaweeds:** Contain iodine—a mineral that regulates and promotes oxygenation of the cells including that of the brain
- **Wheat germ oil:** Rich in octacosanol which helps fight all nerve disorders
- **Jasmine tea:** Helps calm the nerves
- **Turmeric and garlic:** Kill viral infections (many nerve disorders are thought to be caused by viruses) Turmeric contains curcumin which protects the brain tissues

It is a remarkable fact that the elderly living in the villages of India—where turmeric is an integral part of their daily diet—have the lowest incidence of Alzheimer's disease in the world (just one per cent of those above the age of 65 suffer from the disease).

## DEPRESSION

### What

Prolonged unhappiness

### Why

- Chronic stress—the pressure weakens the nerve
- A tragedy
- Imbalance of hormones, especially estrogen
- Birth control pills
- Nutritional deficiencies of iron, potassium, calcium and Vitamin B-complex, especially B12
- As a result of ill health

### Symptoms & conventional treatment

The most common symptoms are fatigue, weakness, insomnia, headache, poor appetite, general disinterest and lack of concentration. In serious cases, depression can lead to suicidal thoughts and, in worst cases, even suicide. Anti-depressants and electric shocks are used as conventional methods of treatments, but not without several side effects. The medication blocks various neurotransmission receptors in the brain leading to endocrinal disturbances, and suppressing the nerves can cause nausea, agitation, headache, dry mouth, blurred vision, drowsiness, dizziness, constipation, skin rash and tiredness. There is also an increased risk of impotence and heart ailments such as tachycardia, cardiac arrhythmia, cardio myopathy and heart failure. If anti-depressants are taken during pregnancy, it can adversely affect the fetus.

## Yogic treatment

- **To remove energy blockages**—maha mudra
- **To increase the healing energy**—suryanamaskara
- **To bring more blood to the brain**—shashankasana, bhumi pada mastakasana and sarvangasana
- **To stabilize hormonal secretion**— kandhrasana, chakrasana
- **To soothe the nerves**—neti and kunjal
- **To de-stress**—kirtan
- **To strengthen the mind**—tratak (although meditation is counter-productive in depression tratak is seen to be beneficial. But it should be introduced after a week or so, and that too with due caution. Its effect should be observed closely. If the condition aggravates, it should be discontinued immediately)

Tyrosine, produced by the thyroid gland, secretes hormones that act as mood lifters. Hence, to treat depression, the treatment of thyroid gland should also be included.

It is important to note that if there's no improvement within a month, conventional medication should be taken simultaneously until the condition improves.

- **Nutmeg:** It works on the cerebral cortex which produces a euphoric feeling

- **Spinach, peas, broccoli, asparagus, milk, cheese and egg:** Rich source of folic acid and Vitamin B12, the deficiency of which can cause depression

- **Wheat germ, onion, tuna, nuts and seeds:** Contain selenium that helps remove copper and lead deposits that can depress the nervous system.

- **Banana**: Contains tryptophan that converts to serotonin, the feel-good hormone

........................................................................................

# FACIAL TICK

## What

Abnormal nerve activity that affects the face.

## Why

- Stress—the constant pressure on the mind can weaken the nervous system

- Nutritional deficiencies, especially of Vitamin B-complex, calcium, and potassium.

## Symptoms & conventional treatment

Involuntary twitching and grimacing are the common symptoms of this ailment. Though facial tick is not a serious ailment in itself, it indicates an abnormality of the nerves. Dopamine blocker is the conventional form of treatment which aims to inhibit the nerves, causing sensitivity to heat and cold, tremor, muscle stiffness, slow movement, dry mouth, blurred vision, and trouble in swallowing. Inactivating the nervous system gradually makes the system weak and ineffective.

## Yogic treatment

- **To de-stress**—mind vision meditation and Om chanting
- **To soothe jumpy nerves**—bhramari pranayama and naukasana
- **To increase the healing energy**—suryanamaskara
- **To send more blood to the brain**—shashankasana, sarvangasana
- **For best tissue rejuvenation**—yoganidra at bedtime
- **Optional addition for faster healing**—single chakra meditation on agnya chakra

## Role of food

- **Milk, sesame seeds, and seaweeds:** These foods are rich in calcium which calms the nerves

Foods to rectify nutritional deficiencies should be included in daily diet.

# INSOMNIA

It is the inability to sleep properly

- Anxiety
- Stress
- Overexcitement
- Excessive intake of tea, coffee or cold drinks
- Certain medication
- Hormonal imbalance
- Hyperthyroidism
- Long-term use of sleeping pills
- Depression
- Nutritional deficiencies of iron, potassium, and Vitamin B-complex

## Symptoms & conventional treatment

Insomnia leads to the degeneration of all body tissues, resulting in some serious illnesses. Barbiturates and benzodiazepines are recommended for treatment, but next day drowsiness—resulting in decreased learning and memory abilities—is a common side-effect of taking the sleep medication. This is because both hypnotic and sedative drugs induce depression of the central nervous system, which decreases the efficiency of all the body parts. Moreover, these drugs suppress very important delta and REM phases of sleep. REM phase, that constitutes 25 per cent of total sleep, is essential for mental health; while during delta phase, that constitutes 50 per cent of total sleep, many vital physical functions—like the secretion of growth hormones, synthesis of proteins, strengthening of the immune system and repair of worn-out tissues—are carried out. Hence prolonged use of these drugs progressively deteriorate one's health; and the immune system becomes weak, exposing the body to all kinds of infectious diseases.

Anti-insomnia drugs depress the respiration centre of the brain, which can make the affected person breathe more slowly and less deeply. This can be harmful for patients with respiratory problems. The drug can also disturb the circadian rhythm, leading to change in metabolism, and also development of problems like gas, constipation, diarrhoea and weight gain.

There is also a direct co-relation between insomnia medication and cancer. According to a study carried out in the US, these drugs increase the risk of cancer by 35 per cent causing five times more deaths than usual. The medication is addictive and it can lead to rebound of insomnia and anxiety. Furthermore, prolonged use of such drugs causes changes in the liver's enzyme pattern, leading to inactivation of all drugs including the sleeping pills.

Even natural sleep-inducing medicines such as tryptophan and serotonin can be harmful. Tryptophan is converted into serotonin—the sleep-inducing neurotransmitter. It was banned by FDA as it created a serious disorder affecting the skin's blood muscles and organs that resulted in severe nerve and muscle pain, beside other problems.

Serotonin can lead to hallucination, tachycardia, sweating, spasms, walking difficulty, while Melatonin reduces the duration of stage 1 sleep.

## Yogic treatment

- **To relax the nerves and induce sleep**—naukasana, ananda madirasana, tratak and ujjayi pranayama in shavasana

- **To de-stress**—internal mantra repetition

- **To induce sleep**—yoganidra and tratak at bedtime

- **Optional addition for faster healing**—single chakra meditation on agnya chakra

## Role of food

- **Banana milk and honey:** It should be taken at night. Banana contains tryptophan that converts to serotonin—the most effective brain relaxant. Honey contains manganese, and milk contains calcium. These help in calming the nerves.

- **Lettuce, peppermint, nutmeg or jasmine tea:** These are rich in lactocarium, which works as a sedative

If you are suffering from insomnia, avoid too much protein intake at dinner. Protein leads to the production of dopamine and adrenaline, which make the brain alert. Amino acid tyrosine found in cheese, red wine, sour cream and yoghurt also has the same effect and should be avoided at night.
According to ayurveda, massaging each sole for 5 minutes with mustard oil at bedtime can prove beneficial. Slow rhythmic music, with a deep pitch, stimulates the body to secrete tranquilizing hormones, and is a natural treatment. Applying nutmeg powder on the eyelids also helps induce sleep. It is also important to stop all activities (that cause anxiety, tension or excitement) 2 to 3 hours before going to bed, because such emotions release adrenaline into the blood stream, making the person feel active and unable to sleep.

# MULTIPLE SCLEROSIS

## What

Inflammation of brain tissues and erosion of their protective lining

## Why

- Virus attack
- One's own immune system attacking the nerves
- Nutritional deficiencies of copper, Vitamin B12 and niacin

## Symptoms & conventional treatment

The most common symptoms are numbness, shivering, weakness, unsteadiness, fatigue, eyesight problems, loss of bladder control and no control over eye movements. People suffering from multiple sclerosis may also experience brief sensation of electric shock, tingling and pain. Corticosteroid, plasma exchange and immune suppressants are usually used for treatment, but not without side effects like liver damage, shortness of breath, high blood pressure, slow heartbeat, blurred vision, and even blood cancer and fatal brain infection. Immune suppressants can lower one's immunity, exposing the body to all kinds of infections.

## Yogic treatment

- **To kill the virus**—amroli (or urine therapy) is considered as the most powerful yogic treatment. Blowing a conch shell can also work as a good substitute

- **To generate heat and inactivate the virus**—bhastrika pranayama
- **To bring healing energy to the brain**—shashankasana
- **To de-stress**—tratak and Om chanting
- **For the best tissue rejuvenation**—yoganidra. at bedtime
- **Optional addition for faster healing**—single chakra meditation on agnya chakra

### Role of food

- **Wheat germ oil, onion, nuts, seeds and tuna:** These are rich in selenium, a mineral needed to make certain enzymes which are deficient in this condition
- **Chicken soup, potato and pulses:** Contain arginine that helps repair worn-out brain tissues and stimulates the growth of T-cells that engulf and destroy the harmful microbes.

## NEURALGIA

### What

Nerve pain

### Why

- Injury, especially if the body is stressed

- Herpes virus
- Nutritional deficiencies of phosphorus, potassium and Vitamin A

## Symptoms & conventional treatment

Brief but extremely sharp painful jabs and excruciating pain are some of symptoms associated with neuralgia. Pain killers, anti-depressants and anti-convulsive medication are used for treatment. Nausea, dizziness, tiredness, difficulty in controlling movements, reduced number of white blood cells, and change in the level of liver enzymes are some of the common side effects. Blurred vision, dry mouth, increased risk of bleeding, shivering, uncontrolled eye movement, weight gain and the inability to pass urine are the other less common side effects.

## Yogic treatment

- **To bring more blood to the brain for healing**—shashankasana and pranamasana
- **To kill the herpes virus**—shankha prakshyalana and blowing a conch
- **To de-stress**—mantra meditation with Om and chanting Om aloud
- **For the best rejuvenation of tissues**—yoganidra at bedtime
- **Optional addition for faster healing**—single chakra meditation—agnya chakra

# PANIC ATTACK

## What

Unexplained paralyzing fear

## Why

- Prolonged stress that weakens the nervous system
- Deficiencies of phosphorus and Vitamin B-complex

## Symptoms & conventional treatment

The common symptoms are extreme anxiety, palpitation, rapid breathing, dizziness, trembling, nervous diarrhoea, perspiration, clammy skin and a choking sensation. Sedatives and anti-depressants can be used to treat panic attacks. The side effects are similar to those experienced by patients undergoing treatment for depression and insomnia.

## Yogic treatment

- **To relax and strengthen the nerves**—tratak
- **To relax and strengthen the mind**—moorcha pranayama
- **To bring more blood to the brain**—sarvangasana
- **To de-stress**—mantra meditation and kirtan
- **For the best rejuvenation**—yoganidra at bedtime

*Yoga and Diet for Ailments*

- **To calm the nerves**—ananda madirasana, naukasana, ujjayi pranayama and bhramari pranayama
- **To calm the mind**— soft music (musical yoganidra is still better)
- **To increase the healing energy**—suryanamaskar
- **Optional addition for faster healing**—single chakra meditation on agnya chakra.

### Role of food

- **Milk, banana and dates:** These calcium-rich foods help calm the nerves and promote sound sleep, that ensures optimum rejuvenation of the nerves.

........................................................................

# PARKINSON'S DISEASE

## What

Degeneration of the brain tissues that control the movements of the body muscles

## Why

- The brain stops producing dopamine—a chemical that transports signals from body cells to the brain cells.
- Nutritional deficiencies of phosphorus and potassium

## Symptoms & conventional treatment

Shaking of the body muscles, inability to control facial expressions, slow bodily movements, stiff limbs, difficulty in speaking, chewing and swallowing, and a stooped and unstable posture are some of the symptoms associated with Parkinson's disease. Drugs to block dopamine inhibitors and chemicals that convert to dopamine are used as conventional forms of medication, but these medicines have many side effects and can be toxic to the heart, central nervous system and the digestive tract. They also inhibit certain secretions, leading to nausea, vomiting, palpitation, arrhythmia, depression, aggression, hallucination and high risk-taking behaviours such as gambling and suicidal tendencies.

## Yogic treatment

- **To arrest brain degeneration**—pranamasana and maha bandha
- **To energize the brain tissues**—bhastrika pranayama and kapalbhati pranayama
- **To relax the brain**—tratak
- **To de-stress**—mind vision meditation
- **For optimum rejuvenation**—yoganidra at bedtime
- **Optional addition for faster healing**—single chakra meditation—agnya chakra

# PERIPHERAL NEUROPATHY

## What

Damaged peripheral nerves

## Why

- Injury
- Poisoning
- Postural defects leading to continuous pressure on the nerves
- Diabetes
- Alcoholism
- Infections
- Nutritional deficiency of Vitamin B-complex especially B2, B6 and B12

## Symptoms & conventional treatment

The most common symptoms are experiencing a tingling feeling, numbness, weakness, unsteadiness and lack of coordination. If left untreated, it can lead to the collapse of the nervous system. Painkillers, anti-seizure medicines and anti-depressants are the conventional forms of treatment, but these medications can cause side effects like nausea, dizziness, drowsiness, constipation and appetite loss.

## Yogic treatment

- **To remove the poison**—detox diet and satkarma (see page 131)
- **To strengthen the peripheral nerves**—namaskarasana
- **To relieve physical stress**—tadasana, bhunamanasana
- **To increase the healing energy**—suryanamaskara
- **To de-stress**—tratak or any other meditation
- **For optimum tissue rejuvenation**—yoganidra at bedtime
- **Optional addition for faster healing**—single chakra meditation on agnya chakra

## Role of food

- **Yeast:** Rich in Vitamin B-complex, should be consumed in sufficient quantities

The diet should be normal but alcohol consumption should be given up.

Diabetics should follow yogic treatment.

· · · · · · · · · · · · · · · · · · · · · · · · · · · · · · · · · · · · · · · · · · · · · · · · · · · · · · · · · · · · · ·

# STROKE

## What

It is the seizure of the brain, leading to immobilization of the body. This happens when either a blood clot blocks the blood flow to the brain or if, due to a ruptured blood vessel, blood supply does not reach the brain tissues. Consequently, the nerve tissues lose their ability to function and eventually they die.

*Yoga and Diet for Ailments*

## Why

- Thickening of blood due to high fat content in it
- Tendency of the blood to clot due to nutritional imbalance
- High stress leading to scarring of the arterial walls, which the body tries to cover with plaque formation. This gradually leads to thickening of the vascular walls which then become rigid, resulting in a rupture
- High pressure of the blood against the arterial walls, leading to its thinning
- A sedentary lifestyle that makes the arteries stiff and brittle

## Symptoms & conventional treatment

Dizziness, sudden weakness, loss of sensation in limbs, double vision, incoherence, slurring and headache are some of the common symptoms. Stroke is one of the largest killers in the world today. In milder form, it can lead to a state of complete or partial paralysis. Conventional treatments like surgery (to remove the blood clot), clot-busting drugs, painkillers and physiotherapy are essential.

## Yogic treatment

The brain tissues, once dead, cannot be regenerated. But yoga can revive and strengthen the weakened living tissues, thus minimizing the problems and preventing further complications.

- **To strengthen the nerves and muscle tissues, and to make the blood vessels pliable**—pawanmuktasana series part 1 is the best yogic treatment for stroke

If the patients are unable to do these asanas properly, they can take help from another person; but gradually, they should be able to do them on their own. Those who cannot move at all, should imagine doing these asana mentally.

- **To clear the energy pathways**—nadisodhan pranayama
- **To exercise and strengthen the brain tissues**—bhramari pranayama
- **To de-stress**—Om Chanting and Om repetition (aloud or mentally)
- **For optimum tissue rejuvenation**—Yoganidra at bedtime
- **Optional addition for faster healing**—single chakra meditation on mooladhara chakra

### Role of food

- **Onion, garlic, turmeric, green leafy vegetables, fish and flaxseed oil:** Lower cholesterol
- **Nutmeg:** Helps in the thinning of blood
- **Yeast, amla, sprouts, and honey:** Improve nerve health

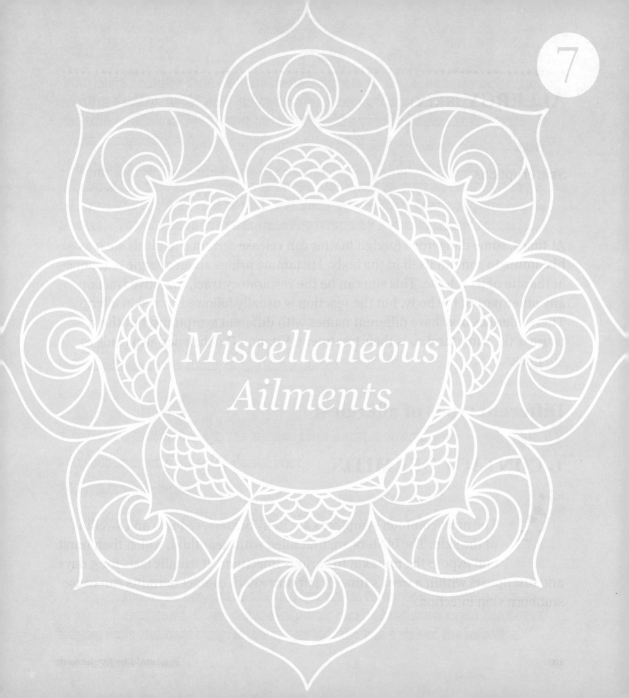

7

*Miscellaneous Ailments*

# ALLERGY (SKIN)

### What

Skin eruptions

### Why

At times, some dangerous foreign matter can release certain chemicals such as histamine to contain itself in the body. Histamine brings about allergic reactions at the site of its release. This site can be the respiratory tract, digestive tract or any other part of the body, but the reaction is usually followed by a skin allergy. These allergies may have different names with different symptoms, but their cause is the same, and so is their treatment. Vitamin D deficiency also leads to allergies.

## Different types of allergies:

# 1. CONTACT DERMITIS

### Symptoms

The most common symptoms are itchy blisters, redness and swelling of the skin. The blisters are first filled with clear fluid, which then burst and expose the raw skin to various infections. It usually lasts for 5 days and disappears within a week's time. If left untreated, contact dermitis can cause stubborn skin infection.

## 2. ECZEMA

Extremely itchy skin, especially behind the knees and the crease of the elbows

## 3. HIVES

Red welts on the skin, often itchy

## 4. URTICARIA

Swelling and redness around the eyes, lips, hands and feet. Sometimes, the throat too is affected which, if severe, can be life-threatening

### Conventional treatment

Anti-histamines and steroids are normally used for treatment of allergies. Histamine is the natural stimulant of the body and anti-histamine is just its opposite. This drug suppresses histamine production in the body inhibiting all functions and leading to a depression in the central nervous system which in turn can cause dizziness, confusion, drowsiness, uncoordinated movement and the inability to concentrate. Continuous depression of the nerves can also lead to mental depression and impaired body functions. The inhibitory effects manifest as dry mouth, blurred vision, nausea, constipation, difficulty in urinating and, in some cases, insomnia, fits, shivering, liver problems, palpitation and other heart ailments. Most patients are advised to avoid the offending allergens; but in practise it is not always possible to do so. This is because the list of allergens is wide and varied, some of the most common being cosmetics, hair spray, shampoo, body lotion, dust, pollen, mold, fungus, smoke, mist, furniture polish, costume jewelry; foods such as egg, shellfish, wheat, corn, berries; and drugs such as penicillin, etc.

## Yogic treatment

- **To settle the disturbed energies**—kunjal for a month and thereafter once every week, for 2-3 months
- **To strengthen the nervous system**—naukasana, trikonasanas
- **To increase the healing energy**—suryanamaskara
- **To normalize the glandular functions**—chakrasana, kandhrasana
- **To balance the energies**—nadisodhana pranayama
- **To stimulate the concerned chakra**—sambhavi mudra
- **To de-stress**—cathartic meditation
- **For optimum tissue rejuvenation**—yoganidra at bedtime
- **To maintain a relaxed state**—Om repetition for 5 minutes frequently; or hundred breaths in shavasana, 3 to 4 times a day
- **Optional addition for faster healing**—single chakra meditation on manipura chakra

## Role of food

- **Omum seeds and jaggery:** Mix ½ teaspoon each and have it twice every day. It helps cure various allergies.

*Yoga and Diet for Ailments*

- **Green gram, black gram, soya bean, and sheep liver:** These contain Vitamin B6, which inhibits excessive histamine production

- **Milk products, oyster, chicken, and peanut butter:** Contain zinc which too inhibits histamine production

- **Brewer's yeast, brown rice, nuts, and cow's milk:** These contain biotin that protects the skin and keeps it healthy

- **Dates and jaggery:** Help fight all skin problems

- **Carrot, nuts, and leafy vegetables:** They are rich in Vitamin A, which is essential for healthy skin

- **Onion, broccoli, cabbage, and alfalfa:** Contain sulfur, also needed for healthy skin

- **Amla and rose hip:** Rich in Vitamin C, which is a potent anti-histamine. Foods rich in Vitamin E and calcium should be consumed since they have anti-allergic properties. Copper-rich foods should also be included in one's diet since it helps reduce histamine.

Drink 4 to 5 glasses of water at the first sign of allergy. The irritating chemicals will be diluted and, in most cases, the symptoms might also subside substantially. Keep drinking water every now and then till there's no swelling.

## ALLERGY (DIGESTIVE TRACT)

### What

It is the distressed reaction of the body to certain foods.

This happens due to the lack of certain pancreatic enzymes that break down proteins into amino acids. The absence of these enzymes leave protein fragments in the system, which the body considers as harmful invaders and attacks. This reaction of body can lead to food allergies.

Pain in the abdomen, diarrhoea, and vomiting are the common symptoms. The allergy can trigger or worsen asthma, eczema and, though rarely, even anaphylaxis (a life-threatening condition).

- **To strengthen the pancreas**—ardha matsyendrasana and gomukhasana

- **To strengthen the liver**—paschimottanasana, dhanurasana, tolangulasana

- **To strengthen the entire digestive system**—part 2 of pawanmuktasana, shankha prakshyalan (preferably the major one) and kunjal

- **To increase the healing energy**—suryanamaskara

- **To relax the nervous system**—ekapada pranamasana and trikonasana

- **To improve pituitary function**— sarvangasana, pranamasana and shashankasana

- **To clear the energy pathways**—nadisodhan pranayama

- **To soothe the nerves**—bhramari pranayama

- **To destress**—cathartic meditation
- **For optimum tissue rejuvenation**—yoganidra at bedtime

**Optional addition for faster healing**—single chakra meditation on manipura chakra.

•••••••••••••••••••••••••••••••••••••••••••••••••••••••••••••••••••

# HIGH CHOLESTEROL

## What

Thickening of blood due to excessive fat content

## Why

- Excessive intake of fatty foods
- Stress, as it does not let the stored fat to be used up

 ## Symptoms & conventional treatment

White streaks on eyelids

If left untreated, high cholesterol can lead to heart attack or stroke

Most anti-cholesterol drugs block the absorption of fat-soluble Vitamins A, D, E, and K. Also, as some of these drugs interfere with liver functions, it can lead to bloating and constipation. They can also deplete an important enzyme essential for heart health. Diabetes is also one of its side effects. Statin (the most common cholesterol-lowering drug), when tested on animals, produced cancer.

## Yogic treatment

As all hormones are made from cholesterol, one needs to improve the glandular health, so that the cholesterol is used up efficiently.

- **To improve pituitary function**—pranamasana and shashankasana
- **To improve thyroid function**—sarvangasana
- **To improve the adrenal functions**—ardha matsyendrasana
- **To improve liver function**—dhanurasana and paschimottanasana
- **To increase the healing energy**—suryanamaskara
- **To improve the vascular health**—part 1 of pawanamuktasana
- **To de-stress**—breath awareness meditation and Om chanting
- **To calm the nerves**—bhramari pranayama
- **To clear the energy pathways**—nadisodhan pranayama
- **Optional addition for faster healing**—single chakra meditation on anahata chakra

## Role of food

- **Garlic and turmeric, especially raw:** These are extremely effective in reducing cholesterol

- **Chaulai, apple, onion, drumstick, drumstick leaves, flaxseeds and fish:** Also lower cholesterol

A low-fat diet is recommended for people suffering from high cholesterol

# FORGETFULNESS (NON-ALZHEIMER'S)

## What

Difficulty in recalling past incidents

## Why

- Drug interaction
- Early sign of cardiovascular disease
- Alcohol intake
- Toxin deposit
- Depletion of Vitamin B12 due to the intake of alcohol and birth control pills
- Diabetes
- Thyroid abnormalities
- Nutritional deficiencies especially of calcium and Vitamin B-complex

## Symptoms & conventional treatment

Inability to recall names faces and past incidents and remember present ones. Vitamin B-complex is generally prescribed to improve the condition.

## Yogic treatment

- **To relax the affected centres of the brain**—veerasana and ananda madirasana

- **To relax and strengthen the brain tissues**—tratak

- **To de-stress**—mind vision meditation

- **For optimum tissue rejuvenation**—yoganidra at bedtime

- **Optional addition for faster healing**—single chakra meditation on agnya chakra

### Role of food

- **Fish, especially sardine:** It contains choline—a nutrient from which acetylcholine (the main brain chemical for memory) is derived

- **Nutmeg powder:** It relaxes the brain tissues

- **Almonds, brahmi, and amla (Indian gooseberry):** These help tone up the brain

# INCONTINENCE

### What

Lack of control over the urinary tract due to muscular weakness

### Why

- Childbirth

- Bladder infection

- Obesity
- Ageing

## Symptoms & conventional treatment

Urine leakage especially while coughing or sneezing, and need for urgent urination are some of the common symptoms. In case of infection, antibiotics are prescribed; otherwise estrogen creams application is recommended.

## Yogic treatment

- **To tone up the urinary tract**—shajoli moolabandha and mahabandha
- **To tone up the muscles of the abdomen**—naukasana
- **To tone up the whole muscular system**—suryanamaskara
- **To lose weight in case of obesity**—dynamic asanas such as suryanamaskar and trikonasana

• • • • • • • • • • • • • • • • • • • • • • • • • • • • • • • • • • • • • • • • • • • • • •

# OSTEOPOROSIS

## What

Gradual hollowing of bones

- Diet deficient in calcium, phosphorus and Vitamin D
- Inability of the body to absorb calcium from the blood, mainly due to hypo-parathyroidism
- Not exposing the body to sunlight
- Sedentary lifestyle

## Symptoms & conventional treatment

Bone ache and loss of height are some common symptoms. In critical cases, the vertebra can break, leading to serious problems. Bone-building mineral supplements are used as medication, but not without side effects like kidney stones, stomach upset, damage of jaw bone, red eyes that are tender and painful, severe bone, joint or muscle pain, and in rare cases, broken leg bones.

Taking calcium without other suitable minerals can make the bones brittle.

## Yogic treatment

- **To strengthen the skeleton**—utthanasana, hasta utthanasana, tadasana, trikonasana, and parvatasana( the 5th step of suryanamaskar)
- **For spinal health and flexibility**—marjari asana
- **For better assimilation of the required nutrients**—part 2 of pawanmuktasana

- **To improve the parathyroid function**—kandhrasana and ujjayi pranayama

- **To increase the healing energy**—suryanamaskara

- **To clear the energy pathways**—nadisodhan pranayama

- **To energize the brain**—kapalbhati pranayama

- **To de-stress**—mantra meditation

- **For tissue rejuvenation**—yoganidra at bedtime

- **Optional addition for faster healing**—single chakra meditation on manipura chakra

 ## Role of food

- **Bone marrow soup**—contains all the nutrients necessary to strengthen the bones

- **Paan (or betel leaves):** It is full of calcium and the mineral is present in a form that is easily assimilated

- **Crab and yeast:** These are one of the richest sources of calcium

- **Chaulai:** It contains all the essential vitamins and minerals

- **Milk, fish, walnut, soya, molasses, sesame seeds, and dark green leafy vegetables:** These should be included in one's daily diet since they are a rich sources of calcium

- **Carrot:** Helps in the absorption of calcium
Apart from calcium, manganese, and phosphorus are also necessary for strong bones.

- **Fish, whole grain, wheat germ, nuts, and sprouts:** Contain phosphorus
- **Green vegetables, apple, wheat germ, corn, and honey:** Rich in manganese
- **Oats:** It contains silica which helps strengthen the bones
- **Alfalfa, yam, and soya:** These contain estrogen which help the bone cells to multiply

Vegetable proteins protect the body from bone loss, thus they should be consumed more than animal proteins.

Avoid white sugar, soft drinks, alcohol, and a high protein diet as these are highly acidic. When the blood becomes acidic, the body tries to neutralize it by releasing calcium—the strong alkaline mineral—from the bones.

Tomato, spinach, beet, cranberry, and chocolates should not be taken since they are rich in oxalic acid which interferes with the process of calcium absorption.

Make sure to sit in the sunlight for half an hour every day.

## TUMOR

### What

A lump of tissues that (unlike cancer) do not invade the neighboring tissues

### Why

- Stress
- Increased acidic content in the body

## Symptoms & conventional treatment

The symptoms depend on the site of the tumor. On the ovaries, it can lead to disturbed menstrual periods; while when in the muscles, it shows as a lumpy growth underneath the skin. In the brain it causes headache, vomiting, weakness, lethargy, uncoordinated movements, and intellectual inabilities. In severe cases, it can damage the nerve cells and may require surgery. But even after surgery the tumor may recur.

## Yogic treatment

As tumors are known to disappear in an alkaline medium, the blood is alkalized by removing toxins by relieving stress from the system, and by taking an alkaline diet.

- **To mobilize the toxin laden lymphatic fluid**—part 1 of the pawanamuktasana series

- **To release the physical tension**—naukasana and shashankasana

- **To soothe the nerves**—bhramari pranayama

- **To increase the healing energy in the body**—suryanamaskara

- **To clear the energy pathways**—nadisodhan pranayama

- **To improve liver function**—bhujangasana and paschimottanasana

- **To burn toxins**—bhastrika pranayama

- **To detoxify the system**—laghoo shankha prakshyalana for five consecutive days and then once every week

- **To de-stress the mind**—any meditation. It should include visualization of the tumor shrinking and disappearing in the end

- **For optimum tissue rejuvenation**—yoganidra at bedtime
- **Optional addition for faster healing**—single chakra meditation on swadhisthana chakra

# URINARY TRACT INFECTION

## What

Infection that affects the urinary tract

## Why

Microbes such as bacteria overcoming the body's defenses in the urinary tract

## Symptoms & conventional treatment

Frequent and painful urination, pus in urine, and fever are some common symptoms associated with UTI. Unless controlled quickly, the infection can spread to the bladder and kidneys with dangerous consequences. Antibiotics can be taken as medication but the problem generally recurs and that too quite frequently.

## Yogic treatment

- **At the first sign of the infection, before fever sets in**—laghoo shankha prakshyalana.

A strong immune system is the best defense against any illness because it can track down all the disease causing invaders and kill them. And to achieve that yoga is extremely effective. *(refer to **Yoga for Busy People** by the same author).*

## Role of food

- **Cumin seeds:** Make an infusion by mixing 2 teaspoons of cumin seeds in 2 glasses of water. Boil this mixture till it is reduced to half. A glass of this concoction should be taken 2 to 3 times every day.

- **Sultana (munakka) and crystal sugar (mishri):** 1 teaspoon of each should be taken twice every day

If the abovementioned foods are taken in the initial stage of the infection, it generally subsides. A diet rich in alkaline content is essential, since such foods alkalize the blood, and throw the infection out.

# VARICOSE VEINS

## What

Enlarged, swollen and progressively thinning veins

## Why

- Malfunctioning valves in the blood vessel
- Obesity
- Long hours of standing

## Symptoms & conventional treatment

Skin ulcers and a visibly enlarged vein with a throbbing, aching sensation are common symptoms. In critical cases, varicose vein can lead to bleeding. Anti-inflammatory drugs and surgery are the conventional forms of treatments; but it has various side effects. Not only is the surgery risky but the problem usually recurs even after surgery (for side effects of the drugs see page 145).

## Yogic treatment

- **To relax the legs**—matsya kridasana
- **To drain out the stagnated blood from the legs**—sarvangasana
- **To improve the health of the blood vessels**—part 1 of the pawan muktasana series
- **To strengthen the blood vessels of the legs**—tadasana and parvarasana (5th step of suryanamaskar)
- **To increase the healing energy of the body**—suryanamaskara
- **To clear the energy pathways**—nadisodhan pranayama
- **To de-stress**—all chakra meditations
- **For the best tissue rejuvenation**—yoganidra at bedtime
- **Optional addition for faster healing**—single chakra meditation on mooladhara chakra

# VERTIGO

## What

Feeling of sudden reeling

## Why

- Disturbed ear fluid that controls the balance of the physical frame
- Infection in the inner ear
- Injury to the balancing centre of the central nervous system

## Symptoms & conventional treatment

Floating sensation and spinning of the head are common symptoms. In severe cases it can cause loss of balance leading to fatal road accidents. Aspirin, dopamine blocker, anti-histamines and antibiotics are used as medication, but not without many side effects.

Aspirin suppresses prostaglandin which stimulates intestinal mobility and its fluid secretions.

As dopamine is the muscle coordinator, its blocking can lead to shivering and involuntary movement of muscles.

Anti-histamines block the protein histamine that makes the body cells work. Its absence can affect all the bodily functions adversely and also lead to headache, drowsiness, and stomach upset.

- **To improve balance**—eka pada pranamasana, natavara asana, and natarajasana
- **To strengthen the nervous system**—trikonasanas
- **To exercise the ear nerves**—shanmukhi mudra and bhramari pranayama
- **To strengthen the nerves of the entire head**—neti
- **To bring more blood to the ears**—pada hastasana and shashankasana
- **To throw out the infections**—laghoo shankha prakshyalan
- **To strengthen the immune system**—suryanamaskara
- **To de-stress the mind**—all chakra meditations
- **For best tissue rejuvenation**—yoganidra at bedtime
- **Optional addition for faster healing**—meditation-agnya chakra

## Role of food

Follow the diet recommended for the nervous system (see page 91).

For better immunity, have an amla and rose hip every day.

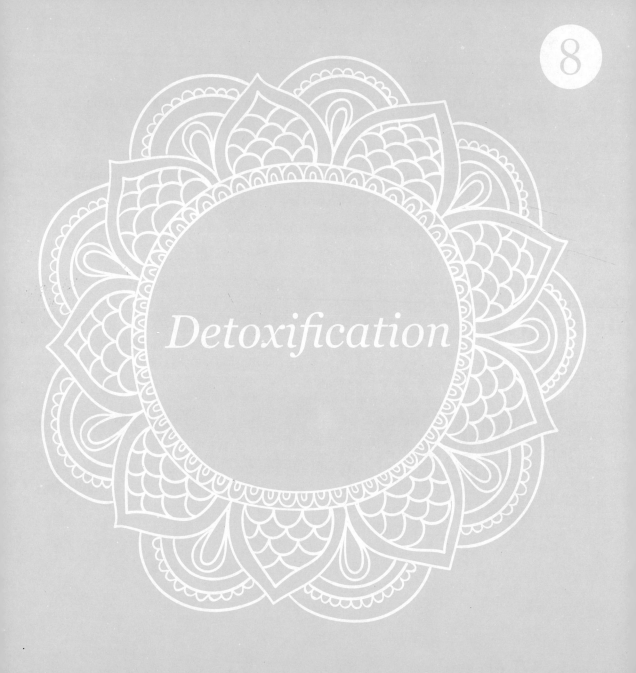

8

Detoxification

Asanas draw a rich supply of blood to a diseased gland or organ to strengthen it. Hence, little can be gained if the blood itself is toxic. In such a condition, the energy generated by asanas and pranayama is used up to burn the stored toxins, leaving hardly any energy for the actual healing. Therefore, it is imperative to detoxify the system while performing yogic practises.

# SATKARMA—THE YOGIC CLEANSING METHODS

There are six cleansing techniques in Hatha Yoga: satkarmas or satkriyas, which are the most effective methods of purifying the system. The best among these six techniques is guru shankha prakshyalan. Within a few hours of practising this, the body eliminates the stored toxins from the intestine and all the tissues. The method involves drinking a huge amount of water prepared in a specific way, practising certain asanas and evacuating the bowel.

Apart from washing the inside of the body clean, guru shankha prakshyalan brings the digestive system to a standstill, giving complete rest not just to the digestive organs but to all the tissues of the body. Such a condition has a wonderful toning effect on the entire system. Even the most sluggish body parts magically revive after this complete state of rest.

Once, a lady from Ahmedabad had come to me with a serious nerve disorder. She had not brought her medical reports, and could not tell me what exactly her diagnosis was. She simply said that her nervous system was failing, and that the doctors in India could not cure her. She was going to America for better medical treatment. I decided to try this great reviver—guru shankha prakshyalan—on her. Her age, condition, and the weather at that time were right for that practice; so I made her do it. Within days, her problem was gone, and has not bothered her since.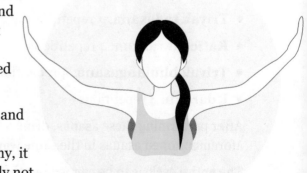

Guru shankha prakshyalan has strict rules and regulations which, if violated, can lead to extremely unpleasant situations. That is why, it should never be done at home, and certainly not without expert supervision. But laghoo shankha prakshyalan, the minor version of this great cleansing kriya, can be done on one's own, as it has very relaxed rules. It may not free the body completely of toxins in one day, as the major one does; but when done regularly over a period of time, it is almost as effective.

## LAGHOO SHANKH PRAKSHYALAN

To be done first thing in the morning.

*Not meant for people with high blood pressure, heart ailments, hernia, and ulcer.*

### Process

Heat 6 glasses of water (it should be hot enough so that you are able to drink it quickly.)

Add 1 ½ spoons of salt in the water and mix it well. Quickly drink 2 glasses of this water and then practise the following asanas:

- **Tadasana**: Repeat 8 times
  It is important to note here that after rising on your toes, here you will need to return to the ground forcefully (banging the heels down)

- **Triyak tadasana**: 4 repetitions

- **Katichakrasana**: 4 repetitions

- **Triyak bhujangasana**: 4 repetitions

- **Udarakh**: 4 repetitions

After performing these asanas, drink 2 more glasses of water and repeat the 5 aforementioned asanas in the same way.

The entire cycle is to be carried out thrice. After you are done, you can relieve your bowels. If you do not feel the urge to do so, walk around on your toes, if possible, and do not sit down. After a while, the water will force the intestine to move faster and you will have the urge to evacuate. After evacuating you should do kunjal. Make sure that you do not eat anything for at least half an hour after kunjal.

Although Yogasanas are done slowly; you need to do them fast for laghoo shankha prakshyalan. The sequence of asanas must not be changed, as it is designed to churn the intestine from the stomach downwards in a specific manner.

## FASTING

Wise men in many ancient cultures incorporated fasting in their traditional rituals, most probably for health benefits. A fast means no work for the digestive organs, which gives them a perfect chance to rest, and repair their own wear and tear. It has been seen that the permeability of the intestine greatly reduces during a fast. Moreover, the energy that would have been used for digestion is now utilized for elimination of toxins.

For thorough detoxification, prolonged fast is necessary. This has to be done in a specific way, since it can harm the body if not done properly. Therefore, long fasts should not be undertaken without expert guidance. But, one can repeatedly observe short fasts of 1 or 2 days, with much benefits. Such fasts can be of the following types:

- **Complete Fast:** Only water is permitted.

- **Juice Fast:** In addition to water, fruit and vegetable juices are also permitted.

- **Partial Fast:** You skip 2 consecutive meals and consume only fruits in the third meal. As fruit is pre-digested, it does not consume the digestive energy. But one needs to choose fruits according to the ailment.

- **Semi-partial Fast:** In this kind of fast, normal food is taken in the third meal.

People with problems of acidity and ulcer must consult a competent therapist before embarking on any of these fasts.

## SPECIAL DETOXIFICATION DIET

The body has its own mechanism to detoxify the system. It first converts the non-water soluble chemicals into water soluble ones, which are then thrown out by the eliminative organs. This change is done with the help of some enzymes, and the enzymes can do the job only in the presence of certain minerals. Therefore, foods containing these minerals must be taken in adequate quantities.

Some of these minerals and their sources are:

- **Copper:** Shellfish, almond, pistachio, whole cereal, mushroom, and gelatin
- **Zinc:** Molasses, mushrooms, wheat germ, pumpkin seeds, prunes, legumes, and fish
- **Magnesium:** All meats and dairy products
- **Manganese:** Nuts, coffee, tea, cereal, and bran
- **Selenium:** Fish, meat, dairy products and unpolished cereals
- **Sulfur:** Onion, broccoli, alfalfa, and cabbage
- **Iron:** All leafy vegetables such as leaves of cauliflower, coriander, and fenugreek

**Other nutrients that help in detoxification are:** beta-carotene, choline, lecithin, and fatty acids. Foods rich in these nutrients are: carrot, papaya, broccoli, cauliflower, zucchini, mushroom, asparagus, lettuce, and other leafy vegetables such as chaulai, bakchoy, celery, and all kinds of fruits.

*Yoga and Diet for Ailments*

**Foods with special attributes that help in the process of detoxification:**

- **Wheat grass juice:** Increases enzymes in the cells

- **Sea weed:** Removes radioactive residues. It also removes lead that can cause depression and mental retardation

- **Apple and orange:** Contain pectin that binds with lead, mercury, and cadmium, facilitating their excretion

- **Garlic:** It is a strong detoxifying agent

- **Coral:** Neutralizes heavy metals and harmful bacteria.( Ayurveda uses this substance in a rose confection called 'gulkand')

- **Jaggery and mint:** Remove harmful chemicals from the blood

- **Green chilli:** Seals cells, preventing permeability of toxins into them

- **Garlic, seaweed, wheatgrass, amla, rose hip, and orange:** Remove aluminum, the metal supposed to cause Alzheimer's disease

## SAUNA

The extreme heat of sauna enters the body through a billion pores and dissolves heavy metals and industrial chemicals. These harmful substances then enter the blood stream and are transported to the eliminative organs via the lymphatic glands to be thrown out of the system.

## MASSAGE

Toxins and cancerous cells are pushed into the lymphatic glands by the body, to be transported to the organs of elimination (the kidneys and the liver). The lymphatic fluid moves only when we exercise or take a massage. Deep massage presses out the stored toxins from the cells to the blood stream, while stimulating the lymphatic system to carry them away for elimination. Massage should follow sauna for best results.

In Ayurveda, various types of medicated oils are used for curing different ailments. But, for general detoxification massages, mustard oil or sesame oil are very good. Mustard oil produces heat in the body which benefits all cold related problems. Sesame oil has cooling properties and it is suitable for summer use. For therapeutic purposes, a daily massage of one hour duration for a month or more is required, while for general detoxification, massaging the body twice a week is sufficient.

## AMROLI

Popularly known as urine therapy, amroli is a potent purifier. To practise it, one needs to take a bland low-protein, vegetarian diet, without any offensive smelling foods such as onion and garlic. For thorough detoxification, only urine and water should be consumed for 2 to 3 days. Thereafter, to complete the treatment and cure the ailment, it is taken thrice a day—the first flow in the morning, an hour after lunch, and again an hour after dinner. Only the mid-stream urine is taken.

After detoxifying the system, care should be taken to maintain this state by periodic cleaning to feel fresh, energetic, and light and prevent all ailments.

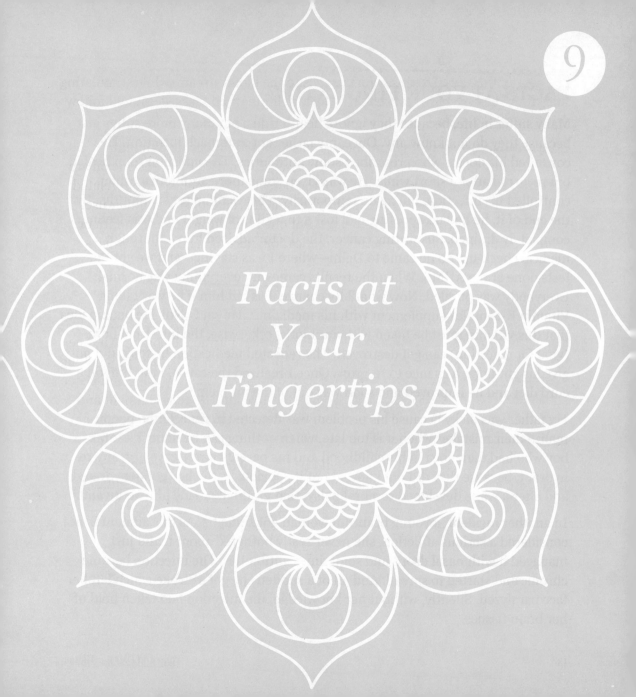

# Facts at Your Fingertips

# 9

# FACTS AT YOUR FINGERTIPS

Many suffer in life, because they ignore health rules; but many more suffer just because they do not know any. Once, my father got a stomach infection. He consulted his doctor who prescribed some antibiotics. The infection soon healed, but recurred after a short while. He was given some more antibiotics; which controlled his infection, but again temporarily. This went on for six months. By the end of it, he had no appetite, had lost 5 to 6 kilos of weight and was feeling completely drained. Suspecting cancer, the doctor advised him a thorough medical check-up. So he came to Delhi—where I was staying—and we got the tests done at the AIIMS. When the results came out, everything was normal. Everybody was puzzled. Now what? By chance, I asked him if he was taking Vitamin B-complex supplement with his medicines. He said, 'No!' He had no idea that this vitamin must be taken with antibiotic, otherwise, the intestinal flora (vital for digestion) can get destroyed. The repeated medication he took, did not give his gut flora, a chance to re-grow. Once I realized the cause, I put him on a curd diet and he improved and soon was out of the problem.

My father was lucky because his problem was detected in time. Often people realize their mistakes when it is too late, when nothing can be done. I know of a boy who had diarrhoea in his childhood and his parents never gave him any re-hydrant, because they did not know about it. Obviously, the boy got dehydrated and after a while developed cerebral palsy, that gradually made him an invalid.

In another incident, a young beautiful woman got sinusitis. As this ailment is not considered a serious affliction, she never really bothered about it and just managed it with nasal drops and sometimes antibiotics. The infection became chronic and started to spread. And all of a sudden she got a stroke which left her face paralyzed. Silently, without her knowledge, the infection had taken hold of her brain tissues.

*Yoga and Diet for Ailments*

To gather knowledge of health is a wise move. Here are some basic important health facts one should know and use in one's daily life.

## pH VALUE

For good health, the blood must remain slightly alkaline. An acid body is a magnet for diseases including some serious ones. In 1931, Dr Otto Warburg won a Nobel prize for proving that the pH value of every cancer patient was extremely acidic. The acid alkaline quotient in the body is measured as pH. A value below 7 is considered acidic and that above 7 is alkaline. It has been seen that at pH 7.45, cancer cells can be controlled and at 8.5 they perish.

Not only cancer cells, but harmful microbes too flourish in an acidic medium and die in an alkaline one. But it is not possible or advisable to keep the pH level too high. One should aim to maintain a pH in the range of 7.4 to 7.5, to prevent all ailments. To achieve that, one should avoid all acid-creating conditions. Some of these include:

- **Stress:** When stressed, the body secretes hormones and gastric juices which are acidic in nature

- **Drugs:** Most drugs are chemicals which irritate the delicate tissues of the inner body, leading to high acid production

- **Pollutants:** Cigarette smoke, gaseous factory wastes, preservatives, additives, and the residue of pesticides and insecticides that are found in food and water are toxic and acidic

- **Shallow breathing:** If one does not breathe out deeply, carbon-dioxide builds up in the body; and since this gas is acidic in nature, it makes the system acidic

- **Too much protein intake:** Proteins need hydrochloric acid for digestion, while the end product of protein metabolism is also an acid, i.e., uric acid. When protein is taken in small quantities, the alkaline juices that are secreted in the pancreas and intestine are sufficient to neutralize the produced acids. But when too much of it is consumed, the body cannot do that properly. Consequently, the surplus piles up, making the system increasingly acidic

- **Fried foods:** These foods are harder to digest and hence remain in the stomach for longer durations, drawing stomach juices that are acidic in nature

- **Red chilli:** It stimulates the stomach to secrete more gastric juices

- **Food containing acids:** Many fruits and vegetables contain various harmful acids such as oxalic acid. Eggs, meat, chicken, oily fish, cheese, white flour, white sugar, cornstarch, cashew nuts, peanuts, sesame seeds, cocoa, coffee, soft drinks, butter, sour fruits, mustard, pepper powder, and soda are examples of some highly acidic foods

The most alkaline kinds of food are almonds, alfalfa, asparagus, cabbage, carrot, celery, and lettuce.

Mushroom, sprouts, ash gourd, bottle gourd, snake gourd, ridge gourd, and all sweet fruits like apple, papaya, banana, pear, and pomegranate are also alkaline.

## IDEAL DIET

While formulating one's dietary chart, it is necessary to keep the following facts in mind:

- **See to it that your diet includes all nutrients.** This is because each nutrient has a specific role to play and cannot be replaced. In its absence, an adverse chain reaction can set in, resulting in serious problems

- **Consuming all nutrients is not enough:** Taking them at the right time is also important, because some nutrients cannot be stored beyond a few hours and one can be deficient in a particular nutrient in spite of taking it regularly. For example, Vitamin B-complex and Vitamin C are water-soluble vitamins that keep passing out of the system all the time, and unless replenished before their exhaustion, there can be a deficiency problem. Similarly, Vitamin A—the resistance builder—gets depleted unbelievably fast during stress. Even the strongest man can have a deficiency of this vitamin within half an hour of being under high stress

- **Food must be well balanced:** Being over-zealous and stuffing oneself with one particular nutrient can be as harmful as the lack of it.
  Here are a few examples:

  - Excess iron can accumulate in the system and create various health problems. In the liver, it can damage this vital organ and cause liver cirrhosis; in the joints, it leads to arthritis and in the heart, it can cause heart failure

  - Vitamin E in excess interferes with blood clotting, leading to excessive bleeding

  - Too much Vitamin C causes nausea, diarrhoea, headache, skin problems, slow healing of wounds, and kidney stones

  - Excess Vitamin B6 can lead to irreversible nerve damage

  - Too much Niacin can worsen diabetes and damage the liver

  - Vitamin A in excess leads to headache, joint problems, liver damage and during pregnancy, it can cause birth defects

As it is difficult and impractical to monitor the quantity of each nutrient, one should eat a wide variety of foods everyday to avoid excesses.

The following is a general guideline that is made on basis of the abovementioned facts:

- Have a yellow fruit or vegetable in every meal

- Have some sprouts every day

- Have a leafy vegetable every day

- Have all the seasonal fruits and vegetables (suitable to your condition) in rotation

- Include some detox items in every meal

- Include some raw food in your daily diet as fruits, salads, sprouts and juices contain enzymes which are easy to digest. Also, they are highly alkaline and ensure better digestion

## EATING RULES

- Food should be hot

- You should eat in silence

- Never fill your stomach fully. Keep at least a quarter of it empty

- Sit for 10 to 15 minutes in Vajrasana after meals

- Walk a 100 steps after that

- Rest for half an hour (lying down on your left side) after lunch

## OTHER RULES

Nutrients should be taken from natural sources only. Synthetic vitamins, minerals, and other dietary supplements can be extremely harmful to the system. They come in concentrated forms, which the body is not used to process, and finds it difficult to handle. It has to exert itself really hard to do so. Secondly, these substances are artificial, and the body perceives everything unnatural as dangerous foreign matter—fit to be discarded. It starts working towards that, which puts even more pressure on the system.

Foods have some other properties too. Some foods heat up the body and dry up the tissues, while some others have a cooling effect and produce extra mucus. Some increase acid in the system while some lead to excessive bile secretion. Therefore, one needs to choose food according to the body's present condition.

The proportion of various kinds of food is also important. A meal should consist of 50-60 per cent roughage, 20-30 per cent carbohydrates, 10-15 per cent proteins, and 5 per cent fat (oil and nuts).

## WATER FACTS

The right amount of water for one to drink is a controversial subject. If too much of it can disturb the electrolyte balance, too little of it can make the blood toxic. A middle path is the best option. So take minimum 6 glasses of water every day and add what you are losing through perspiration.

Also the following recommendations by Ayurveda should be kept in mind:

- Cold water should be taken if one has acidity, does physical labour or in hot weather; while warm water should be taken if the person suffers from cold and cough, jaundice, constipation, gas, indigestion, aversion to food, asthma, tonsillitis, arthritis, fever, and eye ailments.

- Decrease water intake in case of nausea, cold, indigestion, and eye ailments.

- Do not drink water just after or at the beginning of a meal. Also, do not drink water immediately after exercising or evacuating the bowel.

- Drink a glass of water an hour before, and 2 glasses, 2 hours after a meal.

- Do not bathe after a meal.

## FOOD FADS

Every now and then a new theory on food pops up, accompanied by research data to validate its efficacy. Invariably, after some time, another theory emerges, contradicting the earlier one, with equal number of facts and figures to back it. In the meantime, any number of people would have lost their health, and even their lives, following the faulty health advice.

Some popular food fads and their possible consequences are:

- **High-protein no-carb diet:** Claimed as the one that helps lose weight most effectively, it has found many takers who have ended up facing various problems including renal failure. This is because the high uric acid from protein puts excessive strain on the kidneys . Secondly, due to too much protein intake, the system s become acidic, exposing one to the risk of arthritis, gastritis and cancer.

- **No fat diet:** Scared of a heart disease, many people have completely deleted fat from their diet without understanding its full implication. The central nervous system comprising the brain and the spinal cord is made of fat and needs a constant supply of undamaged fatty acids to maintain it. Furthermore, fat keeps the body cells flexible which is essential for proper blood flow, as well as electrical conductivity through the entire nervous system. Not just the brain, no body part can function without cholesterol, because hormones that regulate all the bodily functions are made from this fat. Also, in the absence of fat, the bile flow is not stimulated, which can lead to sediment formation resulting in gall stones. And lastly, the nervous system and the smooth muscles surrounding the alimentary canal (both controlling the peristalsis) become sluggish, leading to constipation and other digestive system problems.

- **Excessive oat bran:** This food supplement is taken to lower cholesterol. With calcium, oat bran can form a compound, the body cannot absorb, and both are expelled out of the body without providing any benefits.

# PROBLEMS OF ALLOPATHIC DRUGS

The fourth killer in the world today, after heart disease, cancer and stroke, is drug abuse. The simplest sounding drug can spell disaster. In 1950s, 23-30 per cent babies were born with limbs and organ defects, just because their mothers unknowingly took anti-convulsive drugs that offered relief from morning sickness.

The effects of some of the common drugs of today are given below.

- **Antibiotics:** antibiotics, as the name suggests, are meant only for bacteria and viruses are not affected by them. But doctors prescribe the medicine indiscriminately for every health problem, and tax the system unnecessarily.

  Antibiotic may kill 99 per cent of the targeted bacteria, but the remaining 1 per cent bacteria (not sensitive to that drug) survive and reproduce a new set of microbes, which become drug resistant, a dangerous trend that has claimed many lives. Furthermore, these drugs lower one's immunity and destroy the intestinal flora affecting the digestive system adversely.

- **Painkillers:** A painkiller can cause a wide range of problems. First, it clings to the intestinal wall and irritates the mucosa that can lead to various gastric disorders such as nausea, vomiting, and indigestion. It also gets absorbed into the mucosa and inhibits the secretions that protect the stomach lining. At the same time, the movement of the digestive tract slows down, which means the drug remains longer in the stomach, and does more harm. This can cause stomach bleeding which has resulted in many deaths. Ulcer can be an outcome.

  Some components of painkillers suppress many antibody-antigen reactions; subdue the bone marrow, leading to less white blood cells, and deplete Vitamin C. All these lower the body's resistance and expose it to all kinds of infections.

  Painkillers reduce the capillary permeability, leading to fluid retention. It also stimulates the sympathetic nervous system, leading to the release of the stress hormone—adrenalin. It interferes with the binding of thyroid hormones which can disturb the metabolism; and it can also lead to increased protein catabolism, resulting in negative nitrogen balance.

Some develop intolerance to the painkilling drugs which can manifest as rashes, urticaria, and spasm in the bronchial pipe.

Lastly, with prolonged use, the body gets used to the existing dosage of the painkiller, calling for higher potency. And these drugs are strong chemicals that can produce a toxic condition, which can cause liver damage and kidney failure. It has been proven that painkillers cause renal damage.

Children below the age of 12 must not be given painkillers as they can cause Rey's syndrome—a fatal condition. For pregnant mothers too, it is not a good idea to take pain killers. It causes the closing of certain ducts connecting to the fetus, leading to serious pulmonary hypertension in the newborn baby. Furthermore, the toxins can enter the fetus' body through the placenta, causing hyperpnoea and bleeding. It has also been seen that many babies whose mothers took painkillers regularly during the pregnancy have hypoglycemia.

- **Anti-inflammatory drugs:** All NSAID (non-steroid anti-inflammatory drugs) are harmful to kidney and liver health. In fact they can cause renal damage even within two weeks of use. They can also cause prolonged bleeding after an injury or surgery. Some common symptoms after taking these drugs are headache, dizziness, confusion, depression, blurred vision, psychotic disturbances, skin rashes, diarrhoea, and dyspepsia.

- **CNS (Central Nervous System) Stimulants:** These drugs stimulate the entire nervous system including the spinal cord. The result can be exhaustion of the nerves, which manifests as headache, shivering, nervousness, irritability, insomnia, confusion, elevated blood pressure, palpitation, etc.

- **Steroids:** The adverse side effects of these drugs are wide and varied. Some common manifestations are hyperglycemia, insulin resistance, diabetes, osteoporosis, cataract, anxiety, depression, colitis, hypertension, immune-deficiency, skin fragility, easy bruising, impaired calcium absorption, negative nitrogen balance, headache, migraine, stunted growth, glaucoma, and cataract. It is also bad for the heart's health as it lowers the good cholesterol (HDL); and the ability to respond to physical stress decreases, which can be dangerous during surgery, trauma, and serious illness.

Female fetus of mothers taking steroids can develop male reproductive organs. With long term use of cortisone, the adrenal gland—which secretes it—starts atrophying, leading to decreased functioning of the pituitary, which in turn affects the functioning of the entire system adversely. Also, it leads to weight gain, loss of bone minerals, muscle weakness, water retention, thinning of the skin, and high blood pressure. Long-term use can even harm the brain.

Inhaled steroid is also harmful as it leads to dryness of the mucus membrane and vascular fragility.

Steroid cream, when used regularly, can lead to skin atrophy.

## POTENTIAL DANGERS OF AYURVEDIC MEDICINE

Sometime back, my uncle took some Ayurvedic medicine for his arthritis. Not only was there no relief from the disease, he started getting fever every day which weakened him so much that soon he was unable to walk and had to be hospitalized. He was diagnosed as having lead and mercury poisoning, and his treating physician said that the medicine that could save his life was available only in the USA. With lot of difficulties, his children managed to get it from abroad and my uncle improved. But he never really recovered. After a long treatment in a reputed hospital in Mumbai, he was discharged. His health remained delicate bringing in various complications and recently he had a blackout, fell down, and passed away.

It was not a stray case. I have myself handled another such case. A lady had once came to me for her ovarian tumor. The tumor disappeared in a month, but soon she felt very unwell. When her blood was tested in the US, it was found to be full of lead, mercury, arsenic and what not—she had tried some Ayurvedic medicine without my knowledge. She consulted me again and I suggested certain yogic cleansing techniques along with some food medicines. After following my advice strictly, she regained her health.

Ayurveda medicine itself is not to be blamed. It is the modern manufacturing process which may be at fault. Ayurveda relies heavily on heavy metals and poisonous substances which in their original form are dangerous for our health. Ancient texts on Ayurveda prescribe elaborate and precise procedures that sometimes take years or even decades to render them harmless and to convert the metals to nano particles that could easily pass through the renal sieve. But today, they are mostly ground and the powdery substance obtained by grinding cannot be eliminated from the system. They accumulate in the body damaging the liver, intestine and the kidneys. According to a research report, sixteen per cent of people in India develop kidney problems and one of the reasons cited was Ayurvedic medicines.

Ayurvedic medicines that are purely plant-based, are safe and effective. Often medicines from our own kitchen are as effective and should be tried first before seeking outside help.

## SOME NATURAL REMEDIES

You can try these natural remedies to prevent the following problems:

- **Cataract:** Pure honey should be applied on the edge of the lower eyelids. When used in the initial stage of this problem, it has often reversed or arrested the process.

- **Chapped lips and heels:** Apply mustard oil in the navel.
- **Cold (in babies):** Make a garland of garlic cloves, crush them a little and put it around the baby's neck. It works like magic.
- **Cuts:** Apply turmeric powder. The cut will heal immediately.
- **Dandruff:** Mix a pack of camphor in two tablespoons of coconut oil (homemade is the best) (see page 279) and apply it on the scalp. Leave it overnight. Next day wash it off, preferably after applying neem decoction.

  Boil a handful of neem leaves in three to four litres of water for 10 to 15 minutes. Keep it on for half an hour. Repeat the process for 2 to 3 days.
- **Gums (to strengthen them):** Take a pinch of salt and add half a teaspoon of mustard oil to it. Dab it on your gums. After the salt melts, massage the gums for 3 to 4 minutes.
- **Hearing loss:** Put a drop of mustard oil in each ear daily.
- **Kidney stones:** Soak a handful of kulthi in a glass of water overnight and drink it in the morning. Repeat this every day. The stone generally dissolves within a month's time.
- **Liver problems:** Take 3 new leaves of a bel (wood apple) tree and eat it every day.
- **Malaria:** Take one basil leaf every day on an empty stomach to prevent it.
- **Marks:** Mix sandalwood paste and turmeric and apply it on the affected area.
- **Nappy rash:** Apply homemade coconut oil.
- **Red eye:** Rose water is extremely soothing. Put a drop in each eye. Small pads soaked in rose water and cooled in the fridge can be put on the eyes for 10 minutes for instant relief.
- **Sty:** Rub your thumb on the opposite palm till it becomes hot, and press it immediately on the sty. Repeat 10 to 15 times. Repeat the whole process as often as possible. The sty would subside in no time.

- **Throat pain:** Crush 3-4 cloves of garlic. Put it in half a cup of hot water; add half a teaspoon of turmeric and a pinch of salt to it. Strain it and sip it slowly.

- **Toothache due to infection:** Rinse mouth with a decoction made from guava leaves. Boil the leaves, till it turns dark. This gives instant relief. People who have used this remedy have not needed antibiotics for root canal treatment. If you chew a guava leaf every day, you will not have any dental infection. If getting these leaves is difficult, then you can try having rock salt mixed in warm water. This is also an extremely effective solution.

- **Wounds:** Homemade coconut oil is a wonder cure. Even diabetic ulcer dries up fast if this oil is applied on the affected area. If that does not work well, bathe the wound with urine. If hesitant to use your own, you can use cow's urine. It is extremely effective. If that too fails, seek medical help as there might be a foreign object lodged in the muscle. A wound must be healed at the earliest or else the infection may spread to the bones, which can be a serious condition.

## NAVEL FIXING FOR BETTER DIGESTION

Indians, mostly in the in rural areas, believe that the control panel of the digestive system, lies behind the navel. They say that if a throbbing is felt directly under the belly button, then everything is fine; and if not, it means the possibility of some kind of digestive disorder. They believe that in the latter case no therapy can be helpful unless the navel is manually 'fixed'. But such one time corrections don't end the problem as the navel has the tendency to slip, unless 'secured' strongly in early childhood.

There are some strange rituals in India, which must have been developed to fix the navel in the childhood for good. One of them, which my mother was also a recipient of, was branding of the side of the navel with the tip of a heated iron tong. My great grandmother, who did that job once a year to every child of the household, never explained the reason for doing so. Perhaps, she herself did not know it; she merely followed a tradition.

Another strange practise—evidently for the same purpose—was to massage a newborn's navel twice daily for a specific period, in a hard circular movement with a cupped hand. The babies would be wailing pitiably, but the massage wouldn't stop. Gradually these practises have died down because of ignorance and the pain it involved.

Most people find it hard to believe in the navel displacement theory. My modern urban mind too, took a long time to do so. But now that I have experienced it many times, I strongly advise everybody to check their navel positioning in case of any digestive problem, and set it right without delay. There are many methods to do that. Below are some simple methods, to be done first thing in the morning on an empty stomach.

## How to Check

- Lie down flat on your back. Keep the arms close to your body with the feet joined and vertical. Ask somebody to see if the 2 big toes are at the same level or not. If not, then the navel is displaced.

- Press your index finger into the belly button and push it down. If you feel the throbbing right at the centre, then the navel is in its place.

- **Only for men:** measure the distance between the navel and your nipples. If the length is the same on both sides, then your navel is in place.

## How to Rectify

- Ask somebody to lift the foot with the shorter toe and placing it on the thigh of the other leg, press the bent knee down to the ground. Hold it there for a while, before lifting the foot and bring it back to its original position. Check again. The process has to be repeated till the toes are of the same length. Then the helper should tie a thread (the thickness of wool) around the neck of the toe. Thereafter, you should sit up straight without taking the support of your elbows. You may take the help from the other person who can pull you up to the sitting posture. Eat some food immediately after this procedure.

- Stand up with the feet together. Lift your arms up and slowly bend forward to touch the toes, keeping the knees straight. Do it 2 to 3 times.

## BODY MOVEMENT

Lymphatic drainage is essential to health. Without it, the tissues are choked in their own toxins and diseases like diabetes, heart ailments, arthritis, and cancer can follow. As the lymphatic system does not have a pump to move the fluid, like the cardiovascular system has, it depends on our body movement to carry the waste away from the cells.

Furthermore, when you do not move, blood circulation slows down, and the body tissues do not get their nourishment fast enough. Exercising for an hour and sitting idle for the rest of the day does not improve the condition. So walk about. Take a 100 steps every half an hour or at least once every hour.

## KEY TO A LONG LIFE

Breathe slow and deep to live long and delay ageing. The body does not age or die according to calendar years; but according to its own usage i.e., how many times your heart has beaten, how many times you have breathed, etc. The slower they are, the longer you live and the longer you retain your youth.

Also, eat less. It slows down the ageing of pineal gland that secretes melatonin, which is essential for slow ageing.

*Yoga and Diet for Ailments*

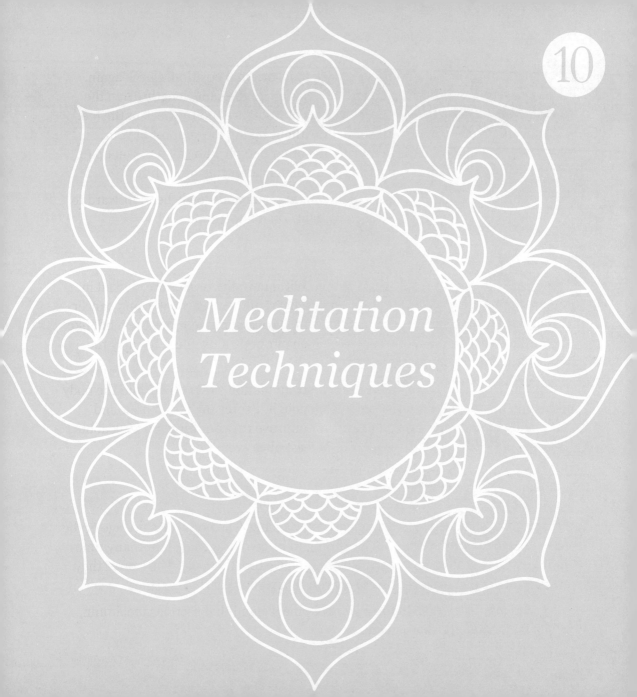

10

*Meditation Techniques*

Outings, shopping or playing games may be pleasurable activities, but they cannot eliminate deep-rooted stress from the system. Moreover, a life without stress cannot be achieved by merely wishing for it to happen. A special technique is required to de-stress the system; and meditation is the most effective and time-tested method to do that. There are innumerable forms of meditation in the world, but you need to choose the right one to get the desired result.

Here are a few things you need to keep in mind before you start practising meditation.

1) **Most forms of meditation require the practitioner to sit in one of the following asanas:**

   - **Sukhasana:** This is the simplest meditative pose where you sit with your legs crossed

   - **Padmasana:** This is the most popular pose for meditation. This asana makes meditation easy by directing the energy from the lower chakras to the highest one

   - **Siddhasana:** Most yogis prefer this pose since it controls the secretion of male hormones

   - **Vajrasana:** People with low back problem, who cannot sit in any of the abovementioned poses for a long time, can meditate in this pose

2) **During meditation, it is necessary to keep the hands in a mudra (hand gesture) to ensure correct energy circuits. You can choose any of the following mudras:**

   - **Gyana mudra:** This benefits the head area

   - **Chin mudra:** Benefits the chest area, especially the lungs

   - **Hriday mudra:** Helps direct energy to the heart

   - **Yoni mudra:** Balances the two hemispheres of the brain and strengthens the nervous system

   - **Bhairav mudra:** Improves concentration and makes meditation easier

Given below are some common forms of meditation that help cure the ailments covered in this book.

# CATHARTIC MEDITATION

Helps eliminate the impression of past traumatic experiences.

- Assume a meditative posture.

- Make sure that your body is straight and still.

- Relax completely by saying 'relax, relax' a few times in your mind, and letting the tension leave the body.

- Move your mind over the body to check if there is still any tension left.

- Visualize your body from the front and try seeing each part in detail. Spend at least a minute in doing so.

- In the same way, visualize yourself from the left, back, right, and again from the front side.

- Now try to listen to a faint distant sound and contemplate on it. *What is making the sound? What must it be looking like? What is it made from? Why are you hearing the sound?* Ask yourself similar questions.

- Then try catching the strains of another sound and think about it.

- Repeat the process in this manner with different sounds.

- After you finish concentrating on a few distant sounds (spend at least 2 minutes in doing so); focus on your breath.

- Just feel the air passing in and out of your nose.

- After half a minute or so pick up another sound which is not too distant.

- Repeat the process with sounds in your vicinity.

- Feel your breath for a minute or so and then let spontaneous thoughts enter your mind. Do not interfere with the thinking process; just be a witness. Pay attention to every thought that strikes your mind. After 2 to 3 minutes, try to block all the thoughts and clear your mind.

- You should feel nothing but blankness. Try to maintain this state for half a minute.

- Again, let spontaneous thoughts come to your mind as before; but now, after thinking these thoughts for a while, discard them with determination.

- Leave your mind free and let more thoughts enter it. Then pick up any particular thought and concentrate on it. Repeat 3 to 4 times.

- Finally, bring to your mind the thoughts of your choice one by one, and work on them. Think of an unpleasant situation you have faced; relive the experience, and then imagine how you would have liked it to be. Do it for 2 to 3 minutes.

- Make your mind blank.

- Now concentrate on a symbol you are comfortable with. It can be a religious symbol; the picture of a deity, saint or your guru; a flower, or a star. Try visualizing it as if it is placed in the space between your eyebrows.

- After a comfortable duration of time, once you start feeling restless, take your mind out to the surroundings. Feel your body, make minor movements, and then open your eyes.

## BREATH AWARENESS MEDITATION

Helps in simple de-stressing.

- Sit straight in a meditative pose with eyes closed.

- Release tension from each body part.

- Concentrate on your breathing process. Ask yourself such these questions: Through which nostril is the air is moving? Is it cool or warm? How thick or thin would it be? How far away from the nose is the air travelling?

- Do this for 1 to 2 minutes. Then just feel the air in your nose for a few seconds.

- Now imagine your breath going from the left nostril up to the space between the eyebrows and coming out from the right nostril; and then re-entering from the right nostril, going up to the same space, and coming out from the left nostril.

- After around a minute or so, imagine your breath to be a silvery form of energy.

- Continue visualizing the alternating breaths for 4 to 5 minutes or so.

- Now imagine your breath entering through both the nostrils simultaneously, going up to the forehead to converge at the same point in between the eyebrows, and then separating and coming out through both the nostrils at the same time.

- Do this step for 4 to 5 minutes.

- Now follow your breath down to the chest.

- Imagine the air flowing from your nose to the chest and your chest to the nose.

- Now count your breath backward from 100 to 0. Count one number, each time you exhale.

Once you reach zero, visualize a symbol you are comfortable with (see Cathartic Meditation), placed in the space between your eyebrows. Concentrate on it for some time till you feel restless.

- Take your mind out to your surroundings, move your body, and then open your eyes.

·· ·· ·· ·· ·· ·· ·· ·· ·· ·· ·· ·· ·· ·· ·· ·· ·· ·· ·· ·· ·· ·· ·· ·· ·· ·· ·· ·· ·· ·· ·· ·· ·· ··

## CHAKRA MEDITATION

Removes the stress that has disturbed the chakras.

- Sit straight in a meditative pose with the eyes closed.

- Feel the contact points between your body and the floor—right foot, right leg, left foot, left leg, and hips.

- Then feel the contact points between your body and your clothes—right leg, left leg, back, abdomen, chest, right arm, and left arm.

- Then feel the air on the exposed parts of your body.

- Now concentrate on your breath by just feeling it in the nostrils.

- Imagine you are breathing to the mooladhara chakra. Your breath enters your body through the point directly in front of this chakra, goes straight to the chakras, and comes out from the same point it had gone in. Visualize your breath in red.

- Repeat mentally the bija mantra 'Lam' of mooladhara chakra along with your breaths. That is, when you breathe in think 'Lam' and again 'Lam' when you breathe out.

- Do this for around 2 minutes.

- Then do the same with swadhisthana chakra. Here the breath should be orange in colour and the mantra, 'Wam'.

- Repeat the process with each chakra, changing only the mantra and the colour

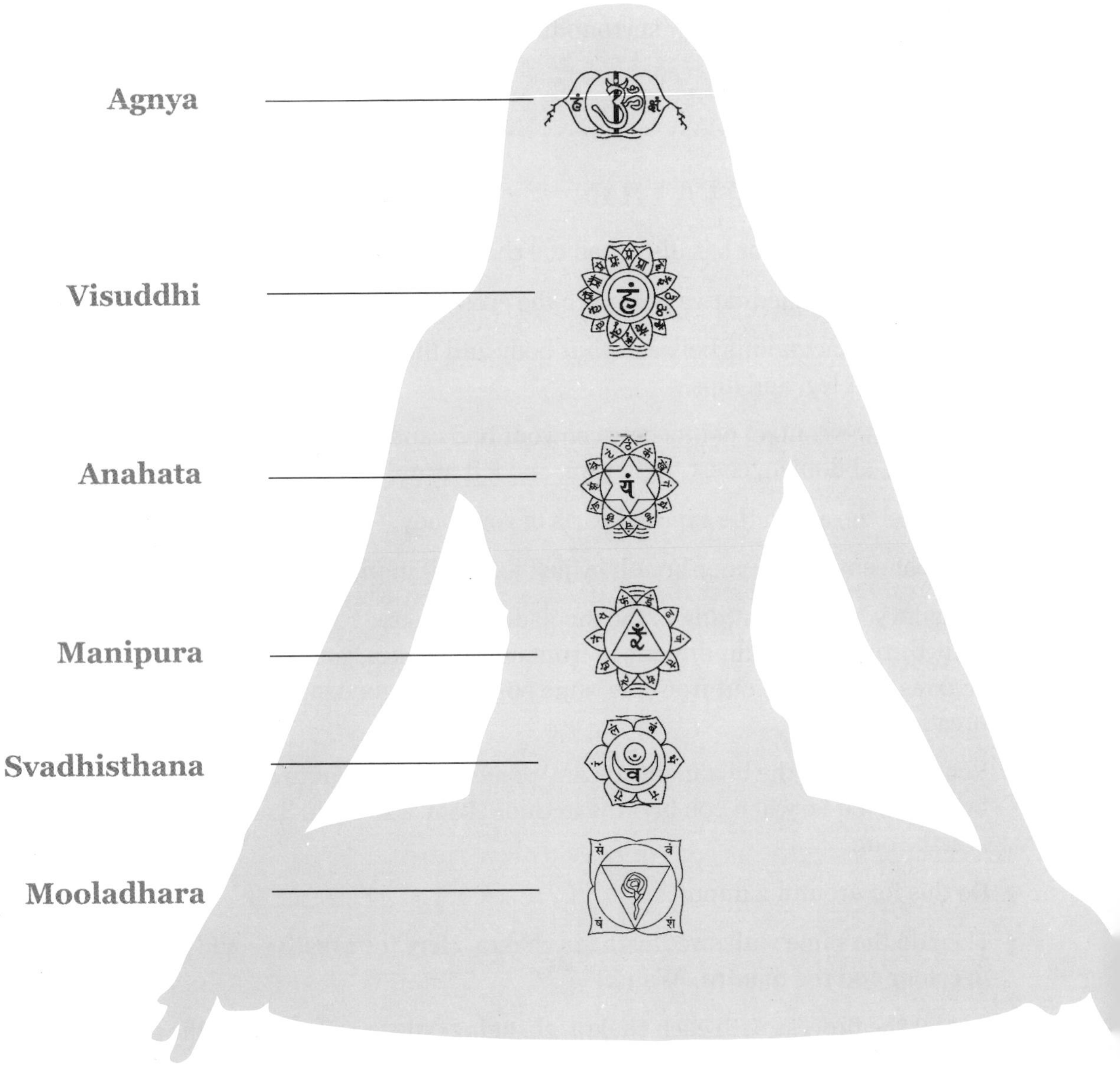

Agnya

Visuddhi

Anahata

Manipura

Svadhisthana

Mooladhara

of the chakra according to the list below:

- **Manipura:** Colour yellow and the mantra is 'Ram'
- **Anahata:** Colour green and the mantra is 'Yam'
- **Visuddhi:** Colour sky blue and the mantra is 'Ham'
- **Agnya:** Colour dark blue and the mantra is 'Om'

- Now take your mind to the base of your spine, and imagine yourself breathing through the spinal cord from agnya to mooladhara.

- As you inhale, your breath rises from the mooladhara to the agnya chakra; and as you exhale, it descends from the agnya to the mooladhara.

- Visualize your breath as golden energy.

- Mentally repeat the mantra 'Om' as you inhale. Repeat 'Om' when you exhale.

- After a while, concentrate on your chosen symbol (see Cathartic Meditation), placed in the space between your eyebrows, for as long as you are comfortable.

- In the end, take your mind out to your surroundings, move your body gently, and open your eyes.

· · · · · · · · · · · · · · · · · · · · · · · · · · · · · · · · · · · · · · · · · · · · · · · · · · · · · · · · · · · · · · · · · · · · · · · · ·

## SINGLE CHAKRA MEDITATION

To activate a sluggish chakra that has led to an ailment.

- Sit in a meditative pose.

- Take a mala of coloured stones (colour of the target chakra to be first determined from the list given in Chakra Meditation) and rudraksh.

- Repeat the bija mantra of the concerned chakra for 5 to 10 minutes.

- This practise should be combined with your main meditation for better healing.

- - - - - - - - - - - - - - - - - - - - - - - - - - - - - - - - - - - - - - - - - - - - - - - - - - - - -

## OM CHANTING

Helps relax quickly.

- Take a deep breath.

- As you exhale say, 'Ooooo' (50 per cent duration of the exhaled breath), 'uuuuuu' (30 to 40 per cent) and then 'mmmm' till you start feeling breathless.

- Practise it for 7, 13 or 27 times.

- Om can also be repeated mentally to keep tension at bay.

- - - - - - - - - - - - - - - - - - - - - - - - - - - - - - - - - - - - - - - - - - - - - - - - - - - - -

## MANTRA MEDITATION

This meditation should be practised with therapeutic (Dhanwantari mantra), longevity (Maha mrtyunjay) or one's personal mantra.

- Sit in any relaxed position.

- Hold a mala of 108 beads in your right hand, keeping the index, ring, and little fingers away from it.

- Rotate the beads and repeat the mantra audibly, mentally, or by whispering. You can also combine all the three modes.

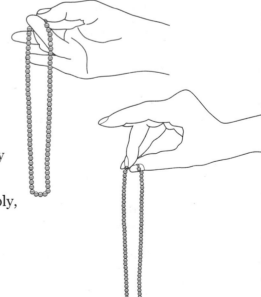

- Do it till you've rotated each bead. It should take around 20 to 30 minutes to complete the mala.

• • • • • • • • • • • • • • • • • • • • • • • • • • • • • • • • • • • • • • • • • • • • • • • • • • • • • • • •

## INTERNAL MANTRA MEDITATION

Helps a person relax deeply and stabilizes his bodily functions.

- Close your eyes, relax the body, and breathe naturally.

- Concentrate on your breath.

- Feel your breath in the nostrils for 2 to 3 minutes; then feel it in your throat by contracting the throat area a little.

- Now imagine, there is a transparent tube between your throat and your navel and your breath moves up and down in that pipe.

- Imagine that when you inhale, it goes up from the navel to the throat; and when you exhale, it moves down from the throat to the navel.

- Continue for 2 to 3 minutes.

- Now add the mantra 'So-ham' to your breath; i.e., repeat mentally 'so' when you inhale and 'ham' when you exhale.

- Practise the mantra repetition for as long as you feel comfortable (ideally 15 to 20 minutes).

- Stop the repetition, and again feel your breath in the nostrils.

- After a minute or so, take your mind out to the surroundings, move your body, and open your eyes.

# MIND-VISION MEDITATION

Helps strengthen the mind and makes it more positive.

- Sit straight in a meditative pose and close your eyes.

- Relax your body consciously by taking the mind to each part and willing it to relax.

- Take a deep breath and as you exhale say aloud, 'Ooouumm...'

- While chanting 'Om' try to feel a resounding vibration in your head.

- Repeat 27 times. (It will take around 6 to 7 minutes).

- After it is done, take your mind into the head and look at the back of the forehead. You will be able to see forms, figures, and colours appearing and disappearing on their own. Just watch them without getting involved. In the beginning, nothing may manifest. Do not bother, just keep a vigil. Eventually they will appear.

- Spend around 10 minutes or so watching these manifestations.

- Concentrate on your chosen symbol (see Cathartic Meditation) for a minute or so.

- In the end, take the mind out to the surroundings, and then moving the body slowly, open your eyes.

# TRATAK

Helps de-stress the mind and strengthens the brain.

- Sit straight in a meditative pose.
- Place the object of tratak (a picture, any object or a lighted candle) in front of you (at eye level and at the distance of one arm length).
- Close your eyes and relax by breathing deep for 1 or 2 minutes.
- Open your eyes and stare at the object without blinking.
- After about 3 minutes (or before if the eyes start to water), close your eyes and concentrate on the after image of the object. It is easier with candle flame, since it creates a strong and lasting visual impression.
- Do this for about 2 minutes.
- If the image fades before time, imagine it placed in the space between your eyebrows.
- Repeat the entire process 2 more times.
- Chant 'Om' 13 times.
- Take your mind out to the surroundings, move about, and open your eyes.

***Note:*** *Candle should not be used for Tratak for more than 1 to 2 months as then its brightness can damage the retina. There are many objects that can be used instead, such as an idol, a flower, an animal, a saint or a guru.*

# RECONSTRUCTION MEDITATION

Promotes regeneration of tissues in a diseased body part.

This practise should be done at the end of any meditative practise.

- First familiarize yourself with the body part you want to reconstruct. Check what it looks like when it is healthy and when it is diseased.

- Visualize the diseased body part.

- Imagine a raging fire engulfing and burning the diseased organ.

- Imagine that the organ disappears and an empty space occupies its place.

- Now visualize a tiny spark of 'prana' (the golden energy) in the centre of that space.

- As you are looking at it, a tiny cell appears inside it.

- The cell is new, healthy, pink, and energetic.

- The cell multiples and so does the spark.

- The cells grow into a full-fledged organ, surrounded by the golden light, which is healthy and pulsating. Slowly the golden light, prana, is absorbed into the organ and you can see the newly built body part.

- Imagine your disease gone and your body functioning superbly.

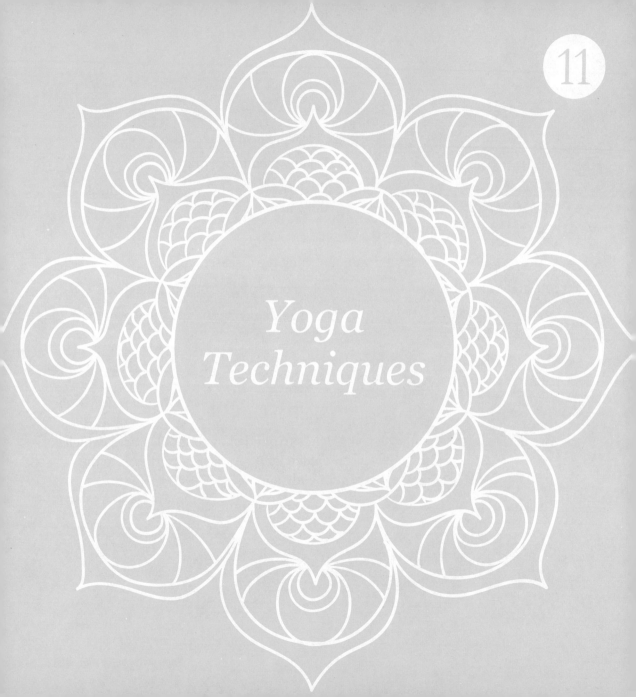

11

# Yoga Techniques

Asanas exercise many muscles of the body; including those that are not frequently used. If the asanas are not done properly, it can lead to soreness and stiffness of these less used muscles. Therefore, if you are a beginner, start your yogic practise slowly; and then gradually advance to the number of repetitions required. Make sure that you do not exceed the prescribed time limit. When doing an asana that requires you to hold a posture for an extended period of time, make sure that another soothing asana follows it.

After selecting the yogic practises, list them as:

- Asana
- Pranayama
- Mudra
- Bandha
- Meditation
- Yoganidra

(Meditation and yoganidra need not be practised with the asanas and pranayamas. They can also be practised separately; but make sure that you practise meditation at the same time every day.)

## SEQUENCE OF ASANAS

Part 1 of pawanamuktasana series, shavasana, part 2 of pawanamuktasana series, shavasana, chakki chalana, nauka sanchalan, namasakara, shavasana, aanandamadirasana, simhasana, veerasana, marjariasana, merudandasana, shavasana, suryanamaskara, shavasana, eka pada pranamasana, natavarasana, natarajasana, akarna dhanurasana, ghutna chalana, dwikonasana, hasta utthanasana, utthanasana, garudasana, vatayanasana, padahastasana, trikonasana, shavasana, sarpasana, bhujangasana, ardha shalabhasana, shalabhasana, dhanurasana, shavasana, sarvangasana, vipareeta karani mudra, halasana, shavasana, matsyasana, shavasana, paschimottanasana, kandhrasana, tolangulasana, supta vajrasana, shavasana, shashankasana, shavasana, sshtrasana, yogamudrasana, bhunamanasana, meru wakrasana, bhumipada mastakasana, shavasana, chakrasana, shavasana, ardha matsyendrasana, gomukhasana, shavasana, matsya kridasana, shavasana.

## Adavasana

- Lie down on your stomach with forehead touching the ground and feet close together.
- Extend your arms above your head.
- Relax the body and breathe normally.
- Do it for 10 to 20 breaths.

*This asana can be done for any duration of time.*

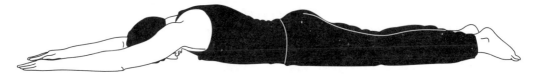

## Akarna Dhanurasana

- Stand with your legs apart.
- Take one step forward (with the right leg).
- Curl your fingers into fists, with the thumbs pressed inside.
- Extend your right arm in front so that it is in line with the right leg (the fist should remain above your eye level).
- Bring the left fist close to the right fist.
- Turn head to look straight towards the right hand.
- Inhaling deeply, pull the left hand back to the left ear while bending the body a little backward.
- Hold this posture for as long as comfortable.

*Yoga and Diet for Ailments*

- Exhaling, again bring your left hand towards the right hand.
- Repeat 5 times on each side.

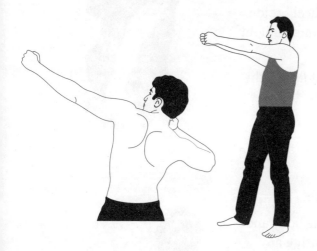
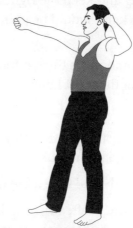
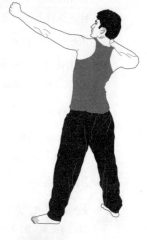

## Ananda Madirasana

- Sit in vajrasana and hold your ankles.
- Look up at the 'V point' in between the eyebrows.
- Take deep breaths and hold this position for as long as comfortable.

*This asana should not to be done if you have a severe knee condition.*

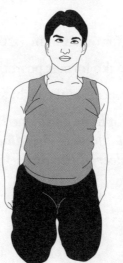
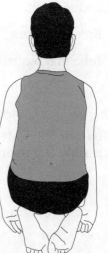

## Ardha Matsyendrasana

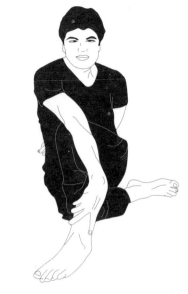

- Sit on the ground with legs stretched out in front.

- Bend the right leg and keep the right heel beside the left hip. (The knee should be pointing straight ahead).

- Bend the left leg and place the left foot flat on the ground in front of the right knee.

- Take the right arm to the left.

- Hitching the right arm with the left knee, hold the left ankle with the right hand.

- Straighten your body and take a breath.

- Exhaling, turn to your left; twisting the body and the head as far as possible without putting any undue strain.

- Breathe naturally for one minute ( 20-30 breaths).

- Inhaling, return to the former position.

- Change legs and repeat on the right side.

*This asana should not to be performed if you are suffering from heart ailments including high blood pressure, stomach ulcer or hernia.*

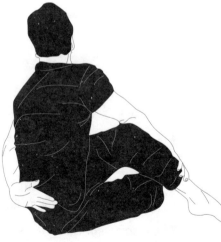

# Ardha Shalabhasana

- Lie down on your stomach with the forehead facing the ground.
- Keep your hands flat under the thighs, with the palms facing down.
- Take a deep breath and lift the left leg.
- Hold this posture for as long as comfortable.
- Exhaling, bring the leg down and repeat with the other leg.
- This completes 1 round.
- Practise 5 to 10 rounds.

*This asana should not be done if you have heart ailments, high blood pressure, stomach ulcer or hernia.*

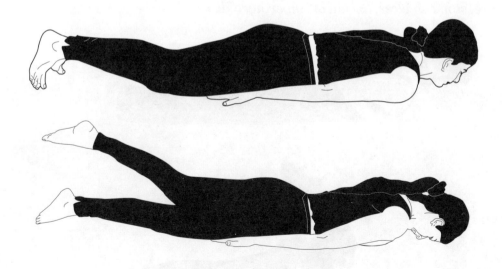

## Bhujangasana

- Lie down on your stomach.

- Keep hands flat on the ground, away from the chest.

- Inhaling, turn your face up and rise to straighten the arms.

- Bend head backward to stretch the neck.

- The back should be well-arched with the lower abdomen touching the ground.

- Hold this posture for as long as you are comfortable.

- Exhaling, return to the starting position.

- Starting with 1round increase the repetitions to 5 rounds.

*This asana should not be done if you have heart ailments including high blood pressure, stomach ulcer, hernia or hyperthyroidism.*

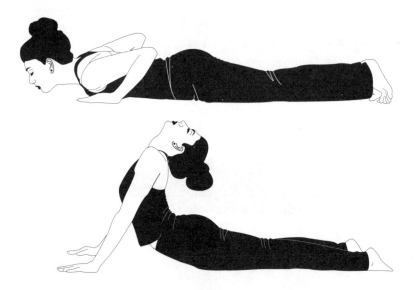

*Yoga and Diet for Ailments*

## Bhu Namanasana

- Sit down with your legs stretched out in front of you.

- Twist your body to the left and place both the hands on the ground (wide apart).

- Exhaling, bend your body to touch your forehead to the ground.

- Hold the posture for around 10 seconds.

- Inhaling, rise and return to the initial position.

- Repeat on the other side as well.

- This completes 1 round.

- Practise 5 rounds.

*This asana should not be done if you have stomach ulcer, hernia or spinal problems and heart ailments including high blood pressure.*

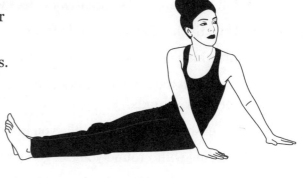

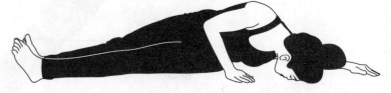

## Bhumi Pada Mastakasana

- Sit with your legs folded under you.

- Placing the hands in front and away from you, lift the body up.

- Lower your head to place it on the ground in between the hands.

- Lift your hips and straighten the legs with the heels together and toes apart.

- Hold the hands behind and lift the toes.

- Breathing normally, hold the posture for as long as comfortable.

- Return to the starting position and place your forehead on the ground to rest for a few seconds.

- Lie down in shavasana while you breathe ten times.

- Starting with 1 round you can go up to 3.

*This asana should not be done if you have heart ailments including high blood pressure; any inflammation or infection in the head area, vertigo, severe eyesight problem, severe asthma, weak back and neck areas or when the blood is toxic.*

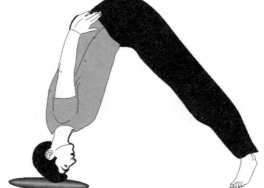

# Chakki Chalana

- Sit down with legs stretched out in front of you.

- Interlock the fingers and hold hands clasped near your abdomen.

- Exhaling and bending forward, move the hands clockwise towards the feet.

- Inhaling, bend backward while still moving the hands clockwise to your body.

- Repeat 10 times.

- Repeat 10 times with the hands moving anti-clockwise.

*This asana should not be done if you have heart ailments, high blood pressure, stomach ulcer, hernia or spinal problems.*

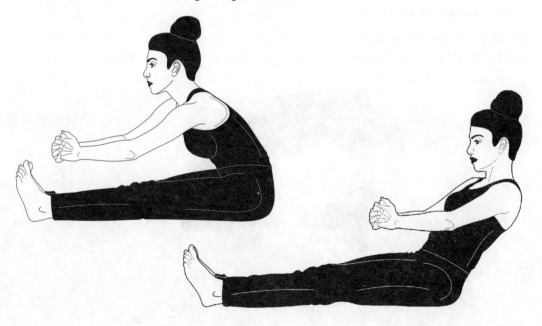

# Chakrasana

- Lie down on your back.

- Bend legs and place your feet beside the hips.

- Place hands beside the neck with fingers pointing towards the body.

- First lift the pelvic, then the shoulder and lastly the head as high as possible to form an arch.

- Breathe normally.

- Hold this posture for 10 to 20 breaths.

- While coming down, first put the head gently on the ground, roll it, then the shoulder and lastly the hip.

*This asana should not be done if you have heart ailments, high blood pressure, stomach ulcer, hernia, weak wrist, spinal problems or when the blood is toxic.*

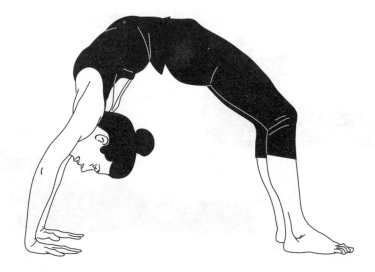

*Yoga and Diet for Ailments*

## Dhanurasana

- Lie down on your stomach with legs apart.
- Bend legs and hold the ankles.
- Inhaling, raise your head and lift the legs up.
- Hold the posture for a comfortable duration.
- Exhale and return to the starting position.
- After 2-3 breaths, repeat.
- Practise 3 rounds.

*This asana should not be done if you have heart ailments, high blood pressure, stomach ulcer, hernia or colitis.*

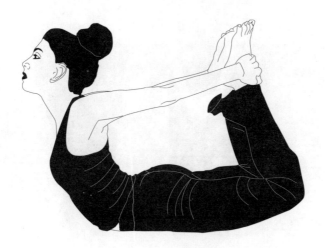

## Dwikonasana

- Stand straight with hands clasped at the back.

- Inhale deeply.

- Exhaling, bend forward while lifting the arms up at the back.

- Inhaling, return to the starting position.

- Repeat 5 times

*This asana should not be done if you have heart ailments, high blood pressure, stomach ulcer, hernia or back ailments.*

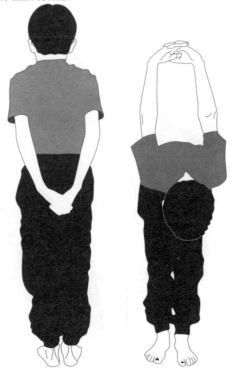

*Yoga and Diet for Ailments*

## Eka Pada Pranamasana

- Stand on the left leg with hands folded in front and the right foot on the left thigh (just above the knee).

- Look straight ahead and take 20 -25 deep breaths.

- Repeat on the right leg.

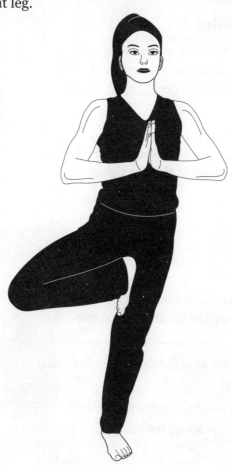

# Eye exercises

*Note: Close your eyes for 30 seconds after each exercise.*

Curl your fingers to make fists. Your thumb should be placed on top of your fingers

## a. Side and center viewing

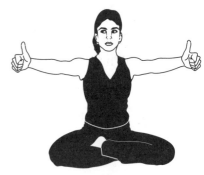

- Stretch your arms in front and move them apart at shoulder level to a position where you can see the right thumb with your left eye and the left thumb with the right eye.

- Look at the right thumb for 3-5 seconds. Then squint to look up at the space between the eyebrows for 3-5 seconds. Lastly, look at the left thumb for the same duration.

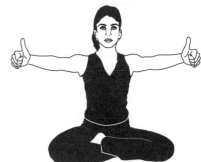

- This is one round.

- Practise 10-15 rounds.

## b. Side viewing

- Stretch your legs in front and keep the left hand on the left leg while holding the right hand in the previous position.

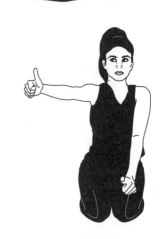

- Look at both the thumbs alternately for 3-5 seconds each.

- Repeat 10-15 times; then change the hands and practise on the other side 10-15 times.

*Yoga and Diet for Ailments*

### c. Rotation

- Rotate your right hand clockwise 5 times and anti-clockwise 5 times.
- Repeat the same with your left hand.

### d. Up and down

- Keep the hands on the leg, with your arms stretched straight.
- Lift the left arm slowly upwards; then bring it down to the left leg while looking at the thumb.
- Repeat 10 times with the left hand and then again 10 times with the right hand.

### e. Distant viewing

- Look at the tip of your nose for 3-5 seconds and then at a faraway object for another 3-5 seconds.
- Repeat 10 times.

### f. Palming

- Close your eyes.
- Rub your palms till they are warm and then place them on the eyelids for 5 to 10 seconds.
- Repeat 10 times.

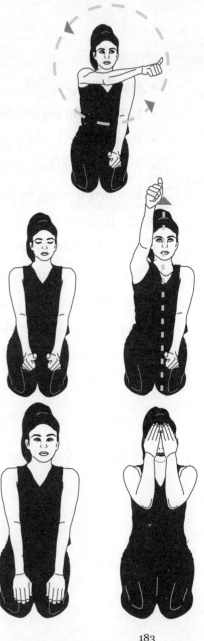

# Garudasana

- Stand straight.
- Lift the right leg and crossing over the left thigh, wrap it around the left leg.
- Keep the top of the right foot on the left calf.
- Entwine the arms and join the hands with the right arm in front of you.
- Lower your body by bending the left knee.
- The right toe should touch the floor.
- Hold this posture for as long as comfortable.
- Straighten up and assume normal position.
- Relax for a while.
- Repeat on the other side as well.

This completes one round. Practise up to 3 rounds.

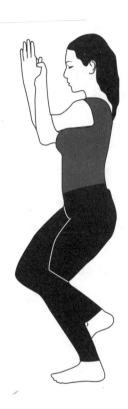

*Yoga and Diet for Ailments*

# Gomukhasana

- Sit down with legs stretched out in front of you.
- Fold the left leg; bring it under the right leg and place the foot beside your right hip.
- Fold the right leg and keep the foot next to the left hip.
- Lift your right arm and bend it backward to point the elbow straight up.
- Take your left arm backwards to hold the right hand.
- Look straight ahead and breathe normally.
- Count your breaths and hold the posture for one minute (20 to 25 breaths).
- Change your position and repeat on the other side for the same duration.

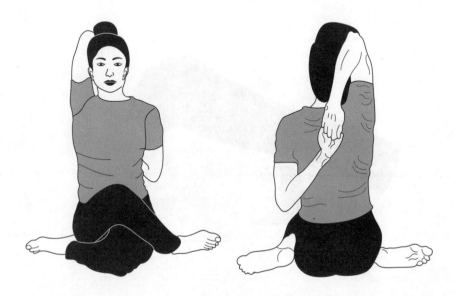

## Halasana

- Lie down with the legs together.

- Take a deep breath.

- Lift legs up and keeping them straight, take them towards the floor (away from the head).

- Breathing normally, hold the posture for as long as comfortable.

- Inhale; and holding your breath, return to the starting position.

- Lie down in shavasana till breathing becomes normal.

*This asana should not be done if you have heart ailments, high blood pressure, hernia, stomach ulcer or back ailments.*

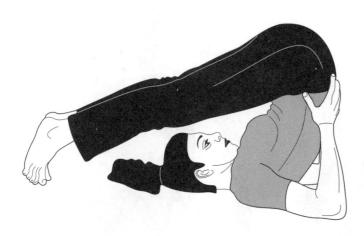

## Hasta Utthanasana I

- Stand with legs apart and hands in front (crossed at the wrists).
- Inhaling, raise arms up, maintaining the position of the hands.
- Turn face up to look at the hands.
- Exhaling, bring arms down to the sides.
- Inhaling, lift them up from the sides and cross the wrists again above you.
- Exhaling, return hands to the starting position.
- Repeat 10 times.

*This asana should not be done if you have heart ailments or high blood pressure.*

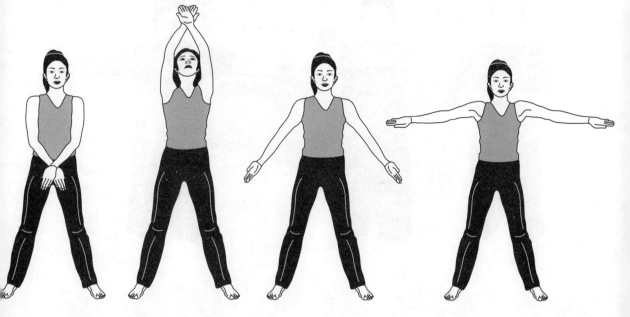

# Hasta Uttahanasana II

- Stand straight with feet together and hands folded in front of you.

- Inhaling, push hands forward and then spread the arms out taking them as far back as possible.

- The arm movement should be similar to swimming.

- Exhaling, bring arms down to the sides.

- Repeat 10 times.

*This asana should not be done if you have heart ailments including high blood pressure.*

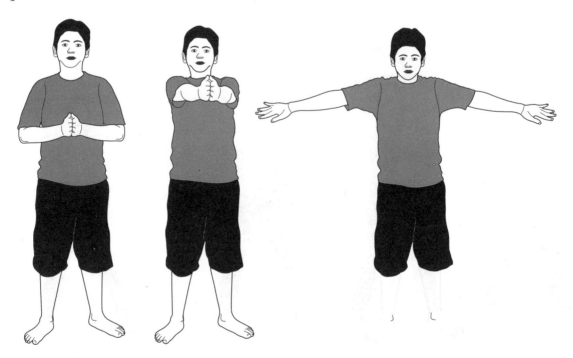

*Yoga and Diet for Ailments*

## Kandhrasana

- Lie down on your back.
- Bend your legs. Keeping the thighs upright, place your feet outside the hips.
- Hold your ankles.
- Inhaling, lift your pelvis up.
- Hold the posture for a comfortable duration.
- Exhaling, come down.
- Repeat thrice.

*This asana should not be done if you have stomach ulcer or hernia.*

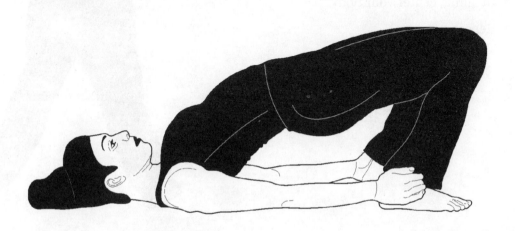

## Katichakrasana

- Stand with legs apart.

- Spread your arms to the sides and take a deep breath.

- Exhaling, turn to your left. Place the right hand on your left shoulder and the left hand on the back of the waist with the palms spread outwards.

- Turn your head and try to look at your heels (over your shoulder).

- Inhaling, return to the centre.

- Exhaling, turn to the right placing the left hand on the right shoulder and right hand on the back of the waist, and look at your feet.

- Inhaling, center your body.

- Repeat 10 times.

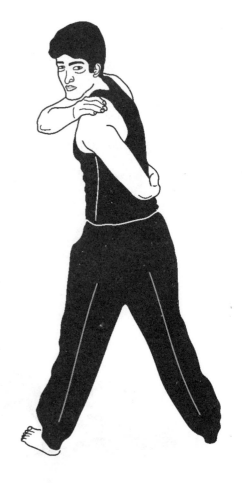

*Yoga and Diet for Ailments*

# Kunjal

- Add 1 teaspoon of salt in four glasses of warm water.

- In the morning, on an empty stomach, drink as much of it as possible.

- Inserting the first 2 fingers in to the mouth, tickle the throat area to induce vomiting.

- The water will gush out.

- Repeat till almost all the water is thrown out.

- Food should not be taken for at least half an hour after doing this practise.

*This practise should not be done if you have heart ailments, high blood pressure, stomach ulcer or eye ailments.*

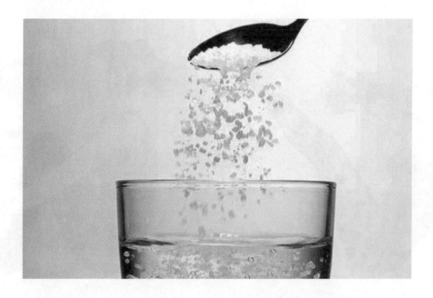

# Merudandasana

- Squat on the floor with feet placed in front of you.

- Hold the big toes and inhale.

- Balancing on the hips, straighten the legs upwards and sideways.

- Hold the posture for as long as comfortable.

- Return to the starting position and exhale.

- Repeat 5 times.

*This asana should not be done if you have heart ailments, high blood pressure or lower back problems.*

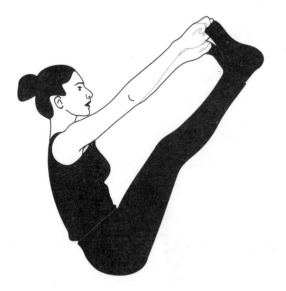
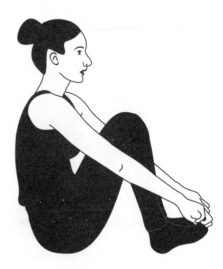

## Marjariasana

- Sit in vajrasana.

- Measure one forearm and one hand length from the knees and place hands on the floor, so that when you rise to your all fours the arms are vertical.

- Move the hands apart so that they are just under the shoulders.

- Inhaling and without moving the arms, bend your head as far back as comfortable, while depressing the back.

- Exhaling, bend head down in front and arch your back.

- The movement should resemble the stretching of a cat.

- Repeat 10 times.

*This asana should not be done if you have heart ailments, high blood pressure or cervical spondylitis.*

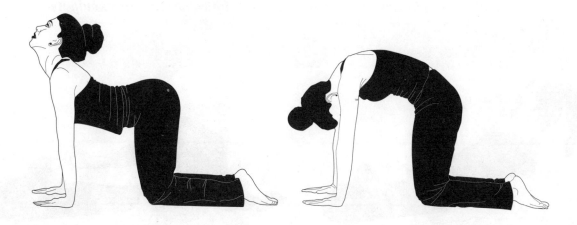

## Matsyasana

- Sit in padmasana.

- Bend backward.

- Supporting the body with the hands and arching the back, lower one side the head towards the ground.

- Hold the toes.

- Breathe naturally.

- Hold the posture as long as you are comfortable.

- If done after sarvangasana, its duration should be half of the former one.

- Rise to the starting position and unlock the legs.

- Lie down in shavasana for 10 breaths.

*This asana should not be done if you have heart ailments, high blood pressure, stomach ulcer, hernia, pregnancy, slipped disc, sciatica or cervical spondylitis.*

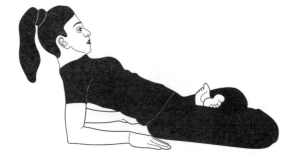
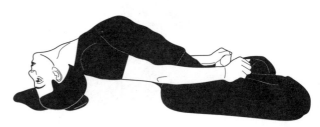

## Matsya Kridasana

- Lie down on your left side with the left arm extended upwards.
- Bend the right leg and keep the knee close to your chest.
- Bend the right arm and place the elbow on the right leg.
- Bend the left arm to hold the hands.
- Make yourself comfortable by turning your body down.
- Keep your left leg straight.
- Breathe normally for 1 minute (20 to 25 breaths).
- Repeat on the other side.

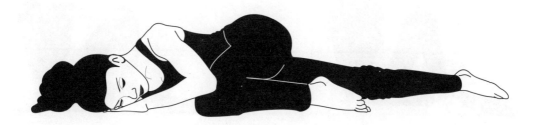

# Meru Wakrasana

- Sit with legs stretched in front of you.
- Place both hands on the floor beside your left hip.
- Looking straight ahead, take a deep breath.
- Retaining the breath in, turn to your left
- Twist your body well and look over the shoulder.
- Hold the posture for as long as comfortable.
- Exhaling, return to the starting position.
- Take a few breaths and repeat.
- Practise the asana 5 times on each side.

*This asana should not be done if you have heart ailments, high blood pressure, stomach ulcer, hernia or a severe lower back problem.*

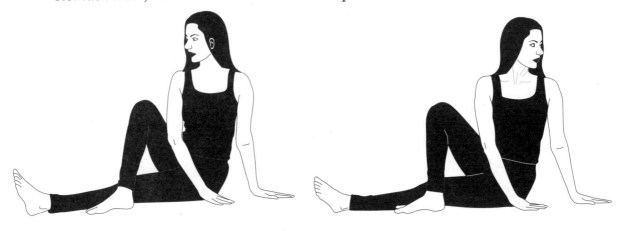

## Namaskarasana

- Squat on the floor.
- Fold your hands and keep the elbows on the inside of your thighs.
- Inhaling, bend your head backwards to look up, while elbowing the legs out.
- Exhaling, bend the head down to the chest, while pushing the elbows in with the legs, and moving the hands forward to straighten the arms.
- Repeat 10 times.

*This asana should not be done if you have cervical spondylitis.*

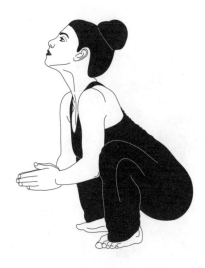
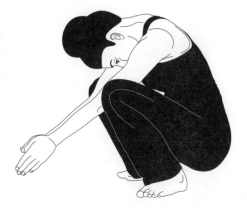

# Nataraj

- Stand straight.

- Lift your right leg and move it towards the left leg.

- Move your right arm to the left and keep it above the leg in a parallel line.

- Join the tips of the thumb and index finger of the left hand and place the wrist above the right wrist with the palm out.

- Breathe normally.

- Hold this posture for a minute.

- Repeat on the other side.

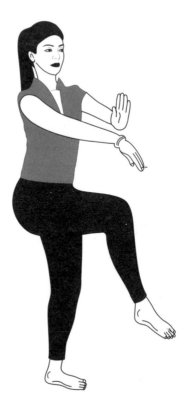

*Yoga and Diet for Ailments*

## Natavara

- Stand straight.

- Lift your right leg and move it towards the left leg.

- Move your right arm to the left and keep it above the leg in a parallel line.

- Join the tips of the thumb and index finger of the left hand and place the wrist above the right wrist with the palm out.

- Breathe normally.

- Hold this posture for a minute (20-25 breaths).

- Repeat on the other side.

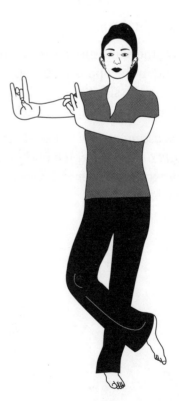

## Nauka Sanchalana

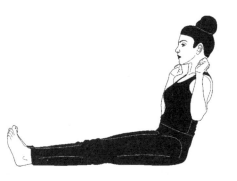

- Sit with your legs joined and stretched in front of you.

- Take a deep breath.

- Close your hands tightly and make fists.

- Exhaling, lift your arms and bend forward (as if you are rowing a boat).

- Inhaling, bend as far back as you can.

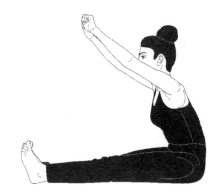

- Repeat 10 times.

- Do the same movement with open palms and in the opposite direction i.e., starting from the sides of your thigh, move them forward and up, then back and down.

*This asana should not be done if you have heart ailments, high blood pressure, stomach ulcer, hernia, colitis or back problems.*

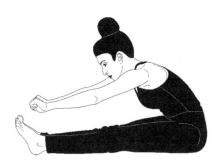

## Neti

- Fill a neti pot with saline water which is slightly above your body temperature (it should taste like tear and feel warm on the wrist).

- Breathing from the mouth (throughout the practise), insert the spout into the left nostril.

- Bend forward and turn the head your right while lifting the pot.

- Water will flow out of the right nostril.

- Empty the pot and remove it while still breathing from the mouth.

- Blow out the nose gently.

- Repeat on the other side.

- To remove water completely, bend forward for a minute; then in that position, tilt your head to the left and to the right for half a minute each.

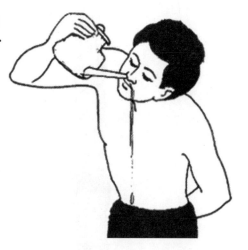

- Lie down in adavasana for a minute and then in shashankasana for the same duration.

- Lastly, dry up the nostrils by doing kapalbhati pranayama.

*Neti should not be done if you have chronic nose-bleeding. Those suffering from heart ailments must seek expert help to do this practise.*

# Pada Hastasana

- Stand straight with the arms raised above your head.

- Take a deep breath.

- Exhaling, bend forward slowly and touch the feet.

- Inhaling, return to the starting position.

- Repeat 10 times.

*This asana should not be done if you have heart ailments, high blood pressure, stomach ulcer, hernia, colitis or back problems.*

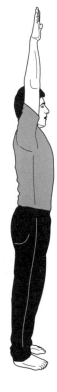
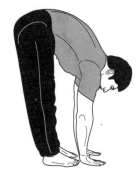

## Padmasana

- Sit with legs crossed.

- The right foot should be on the left thigh and the left foot should be on the right thigh.

- Maintain a straight posture.

*This asana should not be done if you have sciatica.*

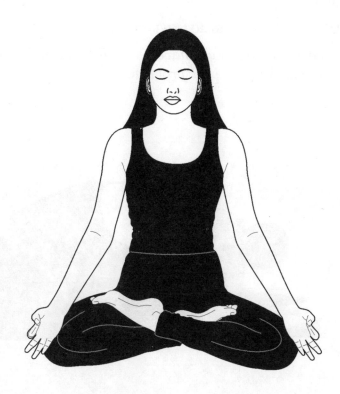

## Paschimottanasana

- Sit down with legs extended in front of you.

- Raise your arms straight up.

- Take a deep breath.

- Exhaling, bend forward and hold your toes (if that is not possible, hold your ankles or your claves).

- Breathe naturally.

- Starting with 5 breaths go up to 20 to 25 breaths.

*This asana should not be done if you have heart ailments, high blood pressure, stomach ulcer, hernia, colitis or back problems.*

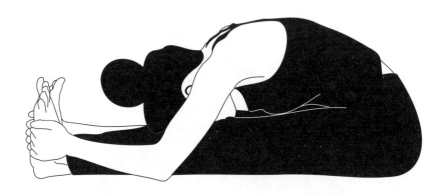

*Yoga and Diet for Ailments*

# Part 1 of Pawanamuktasana series

Sit down on the floor and stretch your legs in front. Keep the hands on the floor behind your body.

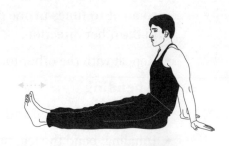

## a. Toes bending

- Exhaling, bend the toes forward; and inhaling, bend them backwards.

- Repeat 10 times.

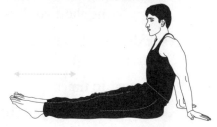

## b. Feet bending

- Exhaling, bend feet forward; and inhaling, bend them backwards.

- Repeat 10 times.

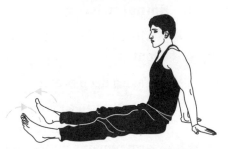

## c. Feet rotation

- Move legs apart.

- Exhaling, rotate the feet forward; and inhaling, rotate them backward.

- Repeat 10 times.

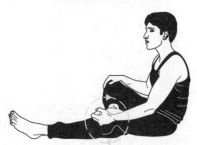

## d. Ankle rotation

- Keep the legs close together.

- Place the right foot on the left thigh; and the right hand on the right knee.

- Holding the right foot with the left hand,

rotate it 10 times in one direction, then 10 times in the other direction.

- Repeat with the other foot.

### e. Leg bending

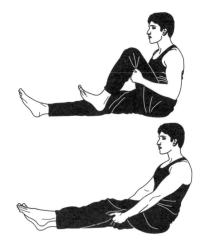

- Hold the right thigh with both hands.

- Inhaling, bend the leg; pulling the knee all the way to the chest, and toes pointing upward.

- Exhaling, straighten the leg with the toes stretched out.

- Repeat 10 times

- Repeat the exercise with the left leg.

### f. Spinal twist

- Move legs wide apart, and stretch your arms out.

- Take a deep breath.

- Exhaling, twist your body to the left and touch the left foot with the right hand while the left arm remains undisturbed.

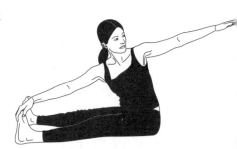

- Inhaling, return to the starting position.

- Repeat on the other side.

- Repeat 10 times.

- The movement should be continuous and in tune with your breathing.

### g. Knee pressing

- Keep the right foot on the left thigh.
- Place the right hand on the right knee and the left hand on the left knee.
- Exhaling, press the right knee down to the floor and inhale as you release it.
- Repeat 10 times.
- Repeat the exercise with the left foot.

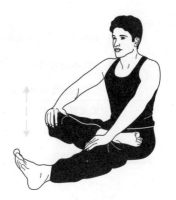

### h. Knee rotation

- Keep the right foot on the left thigh close to the body, and hold the foot with your left hand.
- Hold the right knee with your right hand and while exhaling, rotate the knee down; then inhaling, rotate it upward.
- Repeat 10 times in one direction and 10 times in the other.
- Straighten the legs and relax.
- Do the same with the left knee.

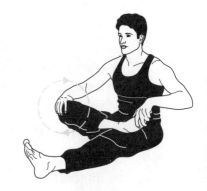

### I. Butterfly

- Bend the legs and join the feet facing each other.
- Holding the feet as close to your body as possible, quickly flap the legs up and down a 100 times.

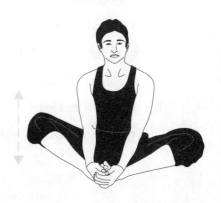

- Breathing should be normal.

- Straighten the legs and relax.

- Sit with your legs crossed (sukhasna) or keep them extended if you are more comfortable in that position.

- Vajrasana also can be assumed if sukhasana is uncomfortable.

## j. Fingers clenching

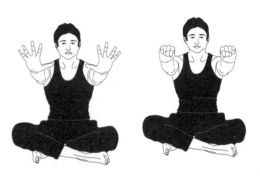

- Stretch your arms in front with the palms facing the wall and the fingers spread out.

- Clench and flex the fingers 10 times, keeping the thumb in when you clench your fingers.

## k. Wrist bending

- Stretch the arms out in front with the fingers pressed together and palms facing downwards.

- Exhaling, bend the hands down.

- Inhaling, bend them upwards.

- Repeat 10 times..

## i. Wrist rotation

- Holding the arms in the same position,

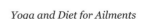

close the hands into fists with the thumbs inside.

- Inhaling, rotate the wrists outwards; and exhaling rotate them inwards.

- Repeat 10 times in one direction and 10 times in the other.

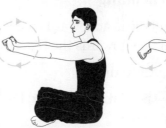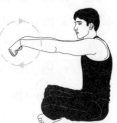

**m. Elbow bending**

- Holding the arms again in the same extended position and palms facing up, take a deep breath.

- Exhaling, bend the arms and touch the shoulders with your fingers.

- Inhaling, straighten them.

- Repeat 10 times.

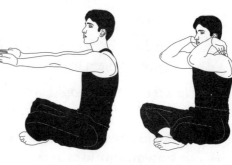

**n. Shoulder rotation**

- Touch your shoulders with the fingers of the respective hands.

- Inhaling, take the arms backwards in a rotating movement; and exhaling, rotate them forward.

- Repeat 10 times in one direction and 10 times in the other.

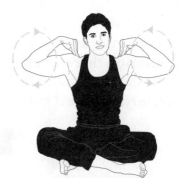

## o. Head bending

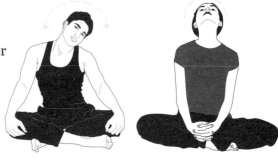

- Bend the head towards the left shoulder and then towards the right shoulder.

- Repeat 10 times.

- Now bend it forward and backward 10 times.

## p. Head rotation

- Rotate the head slowly 5 times in one direction and 5 times in the other direction.

- Lie down in shavasana for 10 breaths, counting them backward.

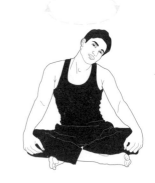

*The last 2 exercises should not be practised by those suffering from cervical spondylitis.*

- **Awareness of 'prana' in pawanamuktasana**

**After each exercise, close your eyes, relax the body and take your mind to the area you've just exercised. Try to locate any unusual sensation there, such as throbbing, tingling, jerking and the likes. Concentrate on the feeling for a while; then open your eyes to perform the next exercise.**

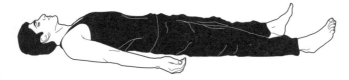

*Yoga and Diet for Ailments*

# Part 2 of pawanamuktasana series

### a. Leg rotation (single)

- Lie down on your back.
- Lift the right leg 6 inches above the ground.
- Rotate the leg 5 times clockwise and 5 times anti-clockwise.
- Bring the leg down to the ground.
- Repeat with the left leg.
- Rest in shavasana for 5-6 breaths.

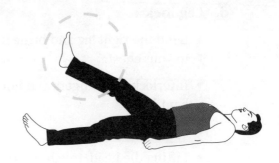

### b. Leg rotation (double)

- Lift both legs together and rotate them 5 times clockwise and 5 times anti-clockwise.
- Rest in shavasana for 5-6 breaths.

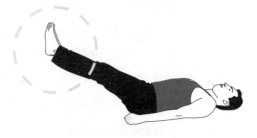

### c. Cycling

- From the same position, lift the legs high up and do the cycling movement.
- First 10 times forward and then 10 times backward.

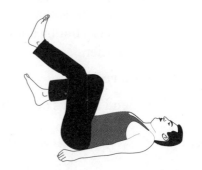

### d. Leg lock

- Bend the right leg and bring it close to your chest.

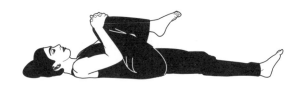

- Interlock your fingers and hold the bent leg.

- Breathe out deeply.

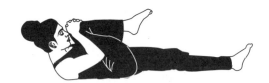

- Lifting the head, touch the knee with your nose while pressing the leg down to the chest.

- Hold this posture for as long as you can hold your breath comfortably.

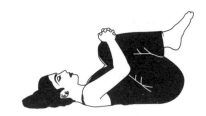

- Inhaling, bend your head down and relax your hold on the leg.

- After a few seconds, repeat the same.

- Practise 5 times with each leg.

### e. Leg lock (double)

- Follow the same steps as the above exercise, but by holding both legs together.

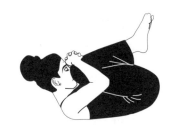

### f. Side rolling

- Bend the legs on to the chest, and

keep hands under your head with
fingers interlocked.

- Roll the lower body from side to side
  while turning the head in the
  opposite direction.

- Repeat 10 times.

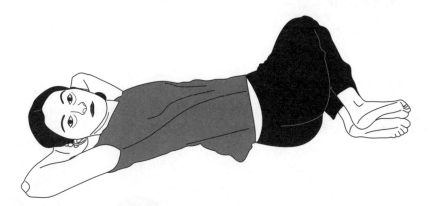

## Naukasana

- Take a deep breath and retaining it, lift your trunk, legs and arms up simultaneously. Hold them about 10-12-inches above the ground.

- The head, hands and feet should be at the same level.

- Hold this posture for as long as you can hold your breath comfortably.

- Exhaling, go down to the floor.

- After 5-6 breaths, practise again.

- Repeat 5 times.

- Relax in shavasana for 10 breaths.

*This asana should not be done if you have heart ailments, high blood pressure, stomach ulcer, hernia, colitis or back problems.*

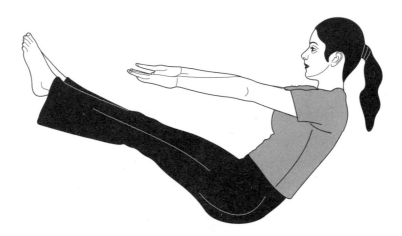

*Yoga and Diet for Ailments*

# Pranamasana

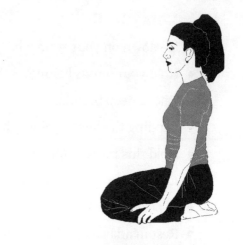

- Fold your legs and sit on your heels.

- Grasp your calves.

- Exhaling, bend forward and keep your forehead on the ground.

- Lift your hips up while rolling the head so that when you are fully raised, the weight of the body falls on the back side of the head and not on the top.

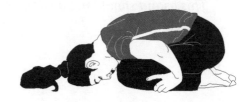

- Hold the posture for as long as comfortable.

- Roll back the head while lowering your body to the heels.

- Inhaling, lift your head and sit up.

- Exhale.

- Lie down in shavasana for 10 breaths.

*This asana should not be done if you have heart ailments, high blood pressure, vertigo or cervical spondylitis.*

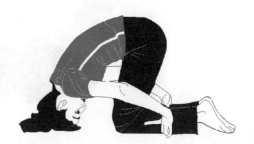

## Sarpasana

- Lie down on your stomach.
- Hold your hands behind.
- Take a deep breath.
- Bending the head backward, rise as high as you can while lifting your arms up.
- Hold this posture for a comfortable duration.
- Exhaling, come down to the starting position.
- Repeat 5 times.
- Rest in adavasana till your breathing becomes normal.

*This asana should not be done if you have heart ailments or high blood pressure.*

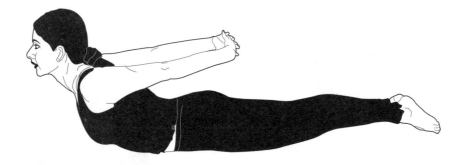

## Sarvangasana

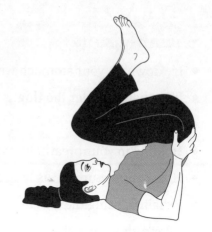

- Lie down on the floor on your back.

- Placing your hands under your trunk, throw the body up to a vertical position.

- The head and shoulder should remain on the ground with the chin touching the chest.

- Breathe normally.

- Starting with 5-10 breaths, gradually increase the number of breaths to 60 or more.

- Add vipareet karani mudra and halasana here if they are a part of your routine.

- Come down slowly to the starting position.

- Lie down in shavasana for 10-15 breaths and then practise an anti-asana such as matsyasana, supta vajrasana , kandhrasana etc for half of the combined duration.

*This asana should not be done if you have heart ailments, high blood pressure, vertigo, cervical spondylitis, if the blood is toxic during pregnancy or in case of enlarged liver, spleen or thyroid.*

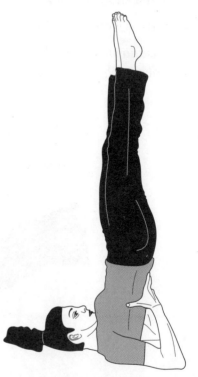

## Shalabhasana

- Lie down on your stomach with the face facing downwards.

- Place hands under the thighs with palms facing down.

- Inhale.

- Holding in your breath, lift your legs together without bending the knees.

- Hold this posture for as long as comfortable.

- Exhaling, bring the legs down.

- After a short rest of 2-3 breaths, repeat.

- Starting with 1 round increase the repetitions to 5 rounds.

*This asana should not be done if you have heart ailments, high blood pressure, stomach problems or ulcer.*

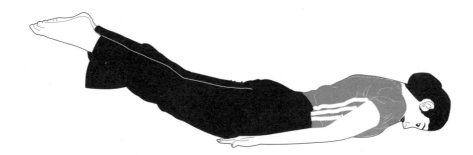

*Yoga and Diet for Ailments*

## Shashankasana (dynamic)

- Sit with legs folded.

- Inhaling, raise your hands up.

- Exhaling and moving your arms with the body, bend forward and try touching the ground with your forehead.

- Hold this posture for a few seconds.

- Inhaling, straighten up to the initial position (with your arms raised).

- Repeat 10 times.

- Lie down in shavasana for 10 breaths.

*This asana should not be done if you have vertigo, slipped disc or cervical spondylitis.*

## Shashakasana (static)

- Practise the same steps as the previous asana; but do it only once, and remain relaxed in the final position for 5 minutes, breathing normally.

- It is important to note that the forehead must rest on the ground and not hang mid-air. If necessary, you may place a few books under the forehead.

*This asana should not be done if you have vertigo or slipped disc.*

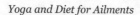

## Shavasana

- Lie down on your back, with the legs around 18 inches apart.

- Move your hands a little away from the body with the palms facing up.

- Close your eyes.

- Breathe naturally.

- Count your breaths backwards with every repetition.

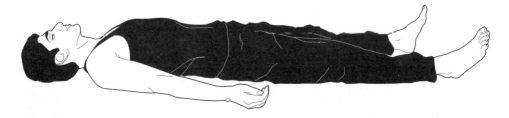

## Siddhasana

- Sit with your legs extended in front of you.

- Bend the right leg and keep the heel pressed against the perineum.

- Bend the left leg and keep the heel pressed against your pubic bone and place the toes in to the fold of the right leg.

- Pull the toes of the right leg up in between the thigh and calf of the left leg.

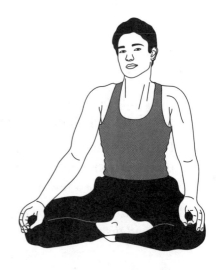

*Yoga and Diet for Ailments*

# Simhasana

- Sit in vajrasana and move the knees apart.
- Keep the hands on the floor, in between the knees, with your fingers pointing inward.
- Bend the head back.
- Cross your eyes to look at the space between your eyebrows.
- Take a deep breath.
- Opening the mouth wide, stick your tongue out.
- As you exhale from the mouth, utter the sound, 'Aaaaaa' till you breathe out completely.
- Repeat 10 times.

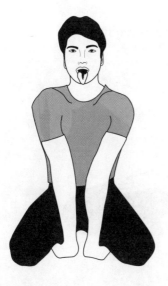
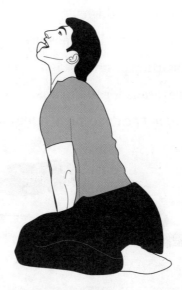

## Sukhasana

- Sit down and simply cross your legs.

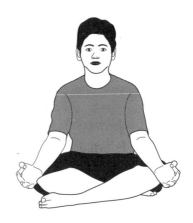

## Supta Vajrasana

- Sit in vajrasana
- Arching the back, and with the support of your arms, bend backward and place one side of your head on the ground.
- Place the hands on your thighs.
- Breathe naturally and hold this posture for as long as required
- Return to the starting position.
- Lie down in shavasana for 10 breaths.

*This asana should not be done if you have any sort of low back problem.*

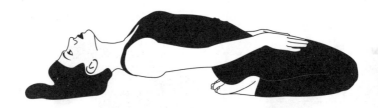

# Suryanamaskar

- 1st step: Stand straight with your feet together and hands folded in a 'namaskar' (greeting) gesture, in front of your chest.

- 2nd step: Inhaling, lift your arms above your head. Turn your face upwards to stretch the neck, and bend a little backward.

- 3rd step: Exhaling, bend forward and place the hands on the floor (a little in front and outside the feet). You may bend the knees initially if necessary.

- 4th step: Inhaling, extend the left leg all the way back and bring the hips down while bending the head backwards. The right knee should be pointing forward.

- 5th step: Exhaling, lift the bottom up and take the right foot back to join the left one putting the head in between the arms (Do not disturb the position of the hands henceforth).

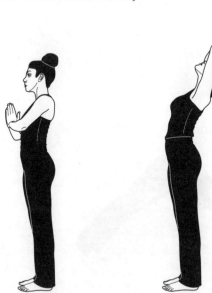
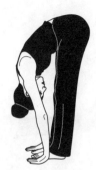

- 6th step: Holding out the breath, lower your body to rest on the ground, but make sure that the bottom is held up and the hands are beside the chest.

- 7th step: Drop the pelvic to the floor, and inhaling, lift your head, then the chest and then the stomach all the way up to straighten the arms. Turn the head up to stretch the neck well.

- 8th step: Exhaling, return to the 5th position.

- 9th step: Inhaling, return to the 4th position.

- 10th step: Exhaling, return to the 3rd position.

- 11th step: Inhaling, return to the 2nd position.

- 12th step: Exhaling, return to the 1st position.

- Repeat on the other side i.e., extend the right leg back.

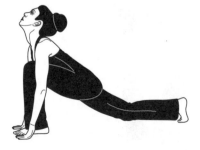
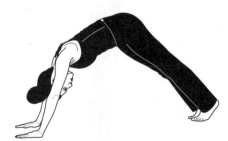

*Yoga and Diet for Ailments*

- These 2 cycles form 1 round.
- Starting with 1 round, gradually increase the number of rounds.
- Practise 6 to 12 rounds according to your capacity.
- Lie down in shavasana till your breathing is back to normal (around 10 breaths per round).

*This asana should not be done if you have heart ailments, high blood pressure, hernia, stomach ulcer or any kind of back problem.*

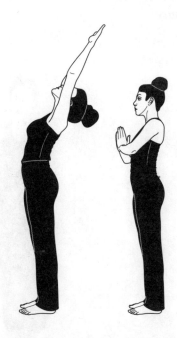

## Tadasana

- Stand straight.

- Interlock your fingers and place them on your head.

- Inhaling, lift your heels and stretch your arms above you (hands turned outwards).

- Turn your face up to look at the hands.

- Exhaling, return to the starting position.

- Practise 10 times.

*This asana should not be done if you have heart ailments or high blood pressure.*

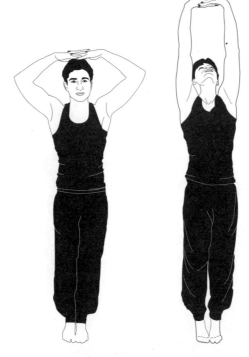

*Yoga and Diet for Ailments*

# Tolangulasana

- Sit in padmasana

- Taking support of the elbows, lie down.

- Keep the hands under your hips.

- Lift both your trunk and the legs while the forearms should remain on the floor.

- Take a deep breath.

- Balancing on the hips, bend head down to press the chin to the chest.

- Hold this posture for a comfortable period.

- Raise your head.

- Exhale and go back to the floor.

- Repeat 5 times.

*This asana should not be done if you have heart ailments, high blood pressure, hernia, stomach ulcer or back problems.*

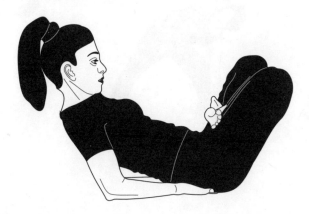

# Trikon I

- Stand with feet apart and arms extended to the sides.

- Exhaling and bending the left leg, bend to the left side and touch the foot with your left hand while turning the face up to look at the ceiling.

- Bring the right arm down to a horizontal position.

- Inhaling, return to the starting position and repeat on the other side to complete a round.

- Practise 10 rounds.

*This asana should not be done if you have heart ailments, high blood pressure or back problems.*

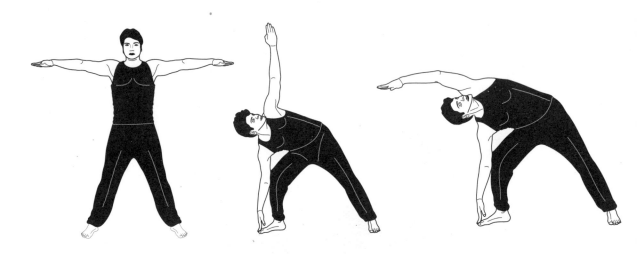

*Yoga and Diet for Ailments*

## Trikon II

- Stand with your feet apart and hands clasped behind.

- Take a deep breath.

- Bend the left leg and exhaling, bend forward to touch the left knee with your nose.

- Inhaling, straighten up.

- Practise on the right side.

- Repeat 10 times.

*This asana should not be done if you have heart ailments, high blood pressure or back problems.*

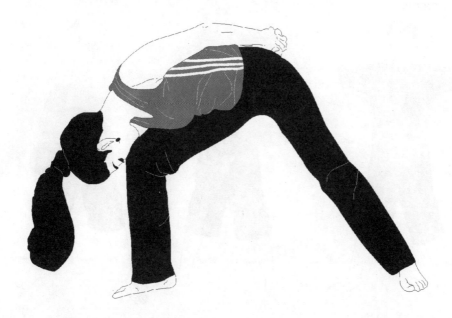

# Trikon III

- Stand with feet apart and arms extended on the sides.

- Exhaling, bend forward.

- Holding your breath, twist the trunk and touch the left foot with the right hand; and again twisting to the other side, touch the right foot with the left hand.

- Return to the bent posture.

- Inhaling, return to the starting position.

- Repeat 10 times.

*This asana should not be done if you have heart ailments, high blood pressure or back problems.*

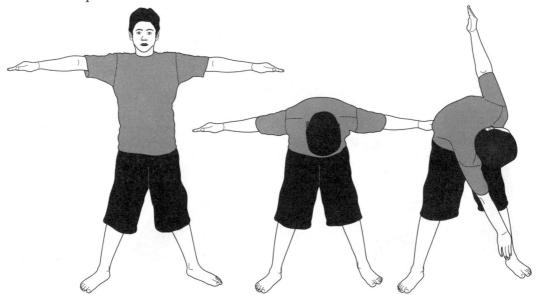

*Yoga and Diet for Ailments*

## Triyak Bhujangasana

- Lie down on your stomach.
- Place your hands on both sides near the chest.
- Keep the face down.
- Inhaling, raise your body (waist onwards) keeping the abdomen firmly on the ground.
- Turn your head to the left to look at your feet over the left shoulder.
- Exhaling, return to the starting position on the ground.
- Practise on the right side.

*This asana should not be done if you have heart ailments, high blood pressure, hernia or abdominal ulcers.*

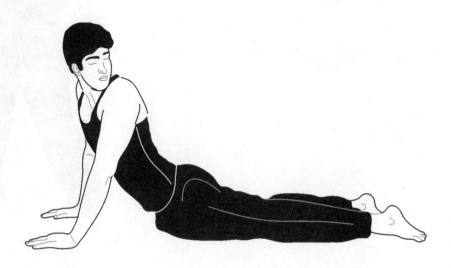

## Triyak Tadasana

- Stand with fingers interlocked.

- Stretch your arms above you and move your legs apart.

- Take a deep breath.

- Exhaling, bend to the left.

- Inhaling, return to the starting position.

- Exhaling, bend to the right.

- Inhaling, return to the starting position.

*This asana should not be done if you have heart ailments or high blood pressure.*

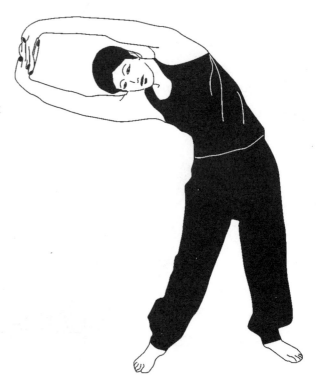

# Udarakh

- Squat on the floor with your hands on the knees.

- Raise the heels and inhaling, turn to your left and put the right knee down on the floor beside the left foot.

- Exhaling, return to the starting position.

- Repeat on the other side to complete 1 round.

*This asana should not be done if you have heart ailments, high blood pressure, hernia or abdominal ulcers.*

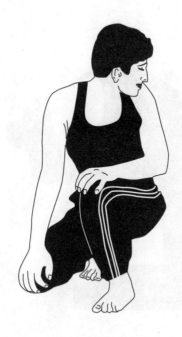

## Ushtrasana

- Stand on your knees.

- Separate the knees so that they are in line with the shoulders.

- Bend backward and hold the ankles.

- The head should be bent as far back as possible without any tension.

- Hold this posture for a few seconds before returning to the starting position.

- Gradually increase the duration and breathe naturally for a minute or 2.

*This asana should not be done if you have heart ailments, high blood pressure or severe back pain.*

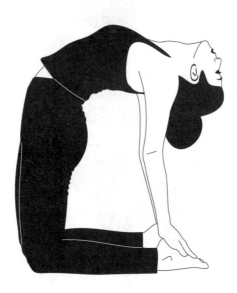

# Utthanasana

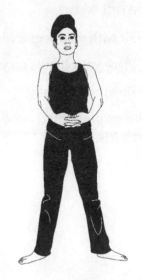

- Stand with your legs apart.
- Interlock your fingers and keep your hands in front.
- Exhaling partially, lower your body a little.
- Inhaling partially, straighten up.
- Exhaling partially, lower your body half way down.
- Inhaling a little, straighten up.
- Exhaling a little, go 3 quarter down.
- Inhaling partially rise.
- Now, exhaling fully, go all the way down; and inhaling, stand up straight.
- This completes 1 round.
- Practise 5 rounds.

*This asana should not be done if you have heart ailments or high blood pressure.*

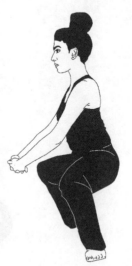

## Vajrasana

- Sit with your legs folded. Your toes should touch each other but not overlap.

- Place your hands on your thighs.

- Breathe normally.

*This asana should not be done if your knee is injured or if you have knee arthritis.*

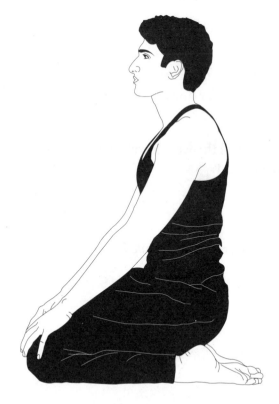

## Vatayanasana

- Stand straight with your feet together.
- Bending the right leg, place it on the left thigh (as high as possible).
- Join hands in front of your chest.
- Take a deep breath.
- Retaining the breath, lower yourself as much as possible (ideally the right knee should touch the floor).
- Breathe normally.
- Hold this posture for a comfortable duration.
- Holding your breath in, stand up.
- Repeat with the other leg to complete 1 round.
- Practise up to 3 rounds.

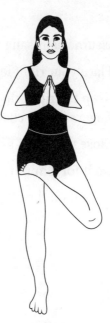

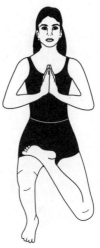

# Veerasana

- Assume vajrasana

- Place your right leg in front.

- Keep the right elbow on the right knee; the palm under the chin; and the fingers on the cheek.

- Close your eyes and breathe normally.

- Do it for a minute.

- Repeat on the other side.

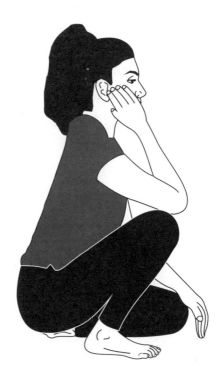

# Vipareet karani mudra asana

- Assume sarvangasana

- Now lower the hips a little so that your trunk makes a 60 degree angle with the floor (the legs should be placed vertically).

- Hold this posture for as long as comfortable.

- Slowly return to the starting position and assume shavasana for 10 breaths.

*This asana should not be done if you have heart ailments, high blood pressure, vertigo, cervical spondylitis, or if the blood is toxic during pregnancy, and in case of enlarged liver, spleen or thyroid.*

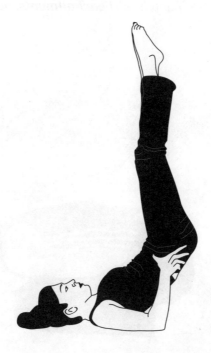

## Yogamudrasana

- Sit in vajrasana.

- Hold the right wrist with the left hand at the back.

- Take a deep breath.

- Exhaling, bend forward and touch the ground with your forehead.

- Breathe normally for a minute.

- Inhaling, rise to the sitting position.

- Lie down in shavasana.

*This asana should not be done if you have heart ailments, hernia and abdominal ulcer.*

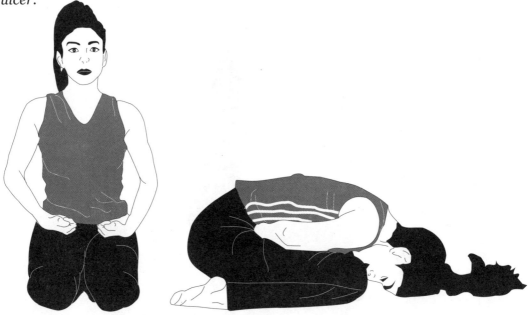

*Yoga and Diet for Ailments*

# PRANAYAMA

## SEQUENCE OF PRANAYAMAS

Nadisodhan, bhramari, sheetli, shitkari, bhastrika, kapalbhati, suryabheda, moorcha, ujjayi.

*Pranayamas should be practised in a meditative pose (except yogic breathing or abdominal breathing).*

## Abdominal breathing

- Lie down in shavasana.
- Inhale deep to first fill the lower part of the lungs, then the middle portion, and lastly the top part.

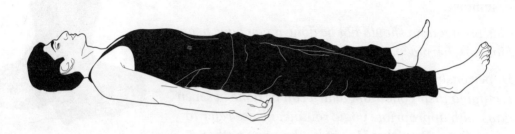

## Bhastrika pranayama

- Sit straight

- Keep the left hand on left knee in chin mudra.

- Place the index and middle finger of the right hand on the forehead, between the eyebrows.

- Close the right nostril with your thumb.

- Breathe rapidly 20 times through the left nostril with force, resembling the movement of a bellow.

- Open the right nostril and close the left one with the ring finger.

- Breathe 20 times from this nostril in the same manner.

- Open both the nostrils and breathe from them simultaneously for 20 times. (Inhalation and exhalation should be equal)

- This completes 1 round.

- Practise 5 rounds in winters and 3 rounds in summer.

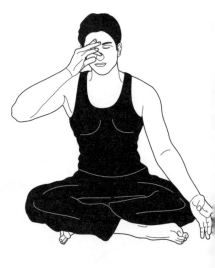

*This pranayama should not be done if you have heart ailments, hernia, gastric ulcers, stroke or epilepsy.*

*Hypertensive people can practise this only after rectifying their condition, which can be done in seven days with appropriate yogic routine. Please refer to **Yoga for a Healthy Heart** by the same author.*

*Yoga and Diet for Ailments*

## Bhramari pranayama

- Separate your teeth and close your mouth over it.
- Plug ears with your index fingers.
- Close your eyes and take a deep breath.
- As you exhale, make a humming sound stretching the breath till you are comfortable.
- Repeat 9 times.

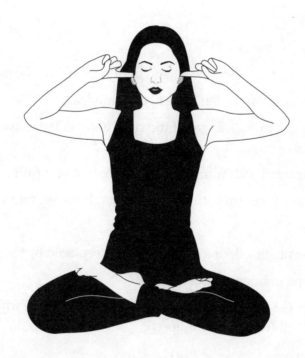

## Kapalabhati pranayama

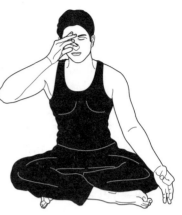

- This pranayama is like bhastrika pranayama, but here the inhalation is natural and the exhalation is forceful.

- Practise 3 rounds.

*This pranayama should not be done if you have heart ailments, high blood pressure, vertigo, epilepsy, stomach ulcer or hernia.*


## Nadisodana pranayama

**1st Stage:** To be practised for a week, and then replaced by the 2nd stage.

- Sit with the left hand on the left knee in chin mudra.

- Place the index and middle finger of the right hand in the space between the eyebrows.

- Close the right nostril with your thumb and breathe naturally from the left.

- Then closing the left nostril with the ring finger, breathe from the right nostril.

- Repeat 10 times.

**2nd Stage:** To be practised for a week, and then replaced by the 3rd stage.

- Assume the same pranayama posture.

- Breathe in from the left nostril. Then closing the left nostril with the ring finger, breathe out from the right nostril.

- Repeat 10 times.

*Yoga and Diet for Ailments*

- Practise from the other nostril in the same way.

**3rd stage:** To be replaced by the 4th stage after a week.

- Assume the same pranayama posture.

- Breathe in from the left nostril and breathe out from the right nostril as before. Then breathe in from the right nostril and breathe out from the left nostril.

- Repeat 10 times.

*This stage onwards, the pranayamas are not meant for people with heart ailments and high blood pressure.*

**4th stage:** Though there are many more advanced stages, this stage will suffice for most ailments.

- Assume the same pranayama posture

- Breathing is similar to the third stage but after inhalation, close both nostrils and retain the breath inside, maintaining the ratio of 1:1:1, meaning -the duration of inhalation, retention, and exhalation should be the same.

- To count both the ratios and the number of rounds, it is convenient to do it in the following manner:

  ♦ Mentally repeat the number of that round, the desired number of times.

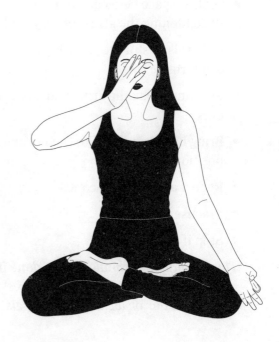

- For example, in the first round, say 'one' 7 times or whatever number you take to complete your inhalation. Then again say 'one' the same number of times, and do the same with exhalation.

- In the second round instead of 'one' say 'two'.

- Continue till you finish till 'ten'.

## Moorcha pranayama

- Fold your tongue and slowly breathe in ujjayi while tilting the head back.

- Look at space between your eyebrows; and straightening the arms, press your knees.

- Hold this posture for as long as comfortable.

- Exhaling, relax the arms and close your eyes.

- Bring back your head to the normal position.

- Repeat after a few seconds.

- Practise 10 rounds.

- Stop if you feel dizzy.

*This pranayama should not be done if you have heart ailments, high blood pressure, brain disorder or weak blood vessels.*

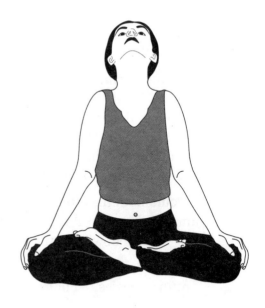

*Yoga and Diet for Ailments*

## Sheetli pranayama

- Sit straight.
- Fold your tongue sideways to form a tube.
- Stick the tongue out and suck the breath in through the tube, making a mild hissing sound.
- Close the mouth and breathe out naturally from the nose.
- Repeat 9 times.

*This pranayama should not be done if you have low blood pressure, constipation or any mucus producing conditions such as asthma or bronchitis.*

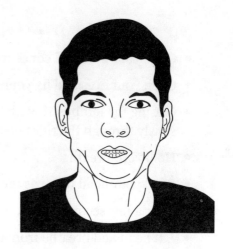

## Shitkari pranayama

- Fold your tongue, close your mouth and tighten your lips.
- Breathe in through the mouth, making a hissing sound.
- Close the mouth and breathe out naturally from the nose.
- Repeat 9 times.

*This pranayama should not be done if you have low blood pressure, constipation or any mucus producing condition such as asthma or bronchitis.*

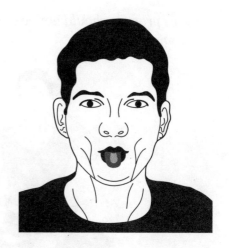

## Surya bheda pranayama

- Close your eyes and concentrate on your natural breathing for a few minutes.

- Open your eyes and fix your gaze on your nose tip.

- Closing the left nostril with the ring finger of the right hand, take a deep breath slowly through the right nostril.

- Hold your breath.

- Bend your head towards the chest and contract the perineum.

- After a few seconds, relax the perineum.

- Lift head and breathe from the right nostril.

- This completes 1 round.

- Practise 3 rounds.

*This practise should not be done if you have heart ailments, epileptics or stomach ulcers.*

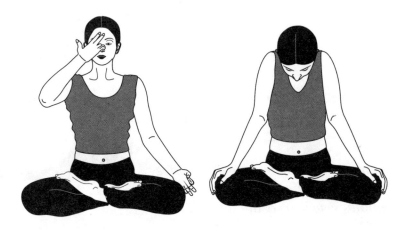

## Ujjayi pranayama

- Fold your tongue and close the mouth.

- Breathe from the nose; and feel the breath in the throat by constricting the throat area a little.

- The breath will make a hissing sound.

- Adjust the contraction, so that you alone should be able to hear the sound.

- Practise 27 rounds.

*This pranayama should not be done if you have low blood pressure or slow heartbeat.*

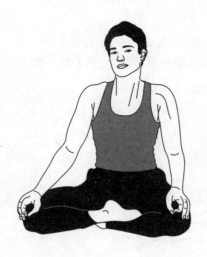

# MUDRA

## Ashwini mudra

- Sit on the floor and cross your legs.
- Inhale and retaining the breath, contract the sphincter muscles and hold it for a few seconds.
- Breathe out while releasing the contraction.
- Relax for a few seconds and then repeat.
- Practise 50 times.
- This mudra can also be done faster without breath retention.

*This mudra should not be done if you have fistula.*

## Bhairav mudra

- Keep your hands on the lap with the right hand on top of the left.
- The palms should be facing up.

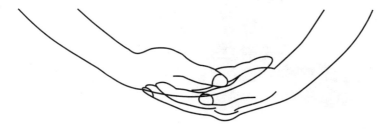

## Chin mudra

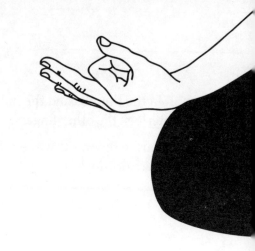

- Touch the base of the thumb with the tip of the index finger and keep the hand on the knee with the palm facing up.

## Bhoochari mudra

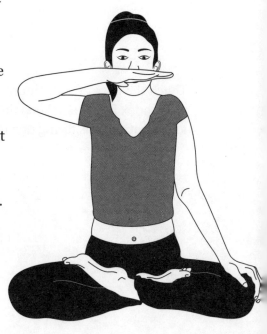

- Sit straight in padmasana with left hand on the left knee in gyana mudra.

- Close your eyes and relax.

- Open the eyes and lift the right hand to the face with your palm facing downwards and the elbow pointing outwards.

- Placing the thumb's nail under the nose, gaze at the tip of the little finger without blinking.

- After 1 minute, remove your hand; but keep gazing at the same point for as long as possible.

- Continue practising for 4-5 minutes.

- Breathing should be natural.

*This mudra should not be done if you have glaucoma, retinopathy or if you recently had an eye surgery.*

## Yoni mudra

- Join the thumbs and the index fingers and interlock the other fingers.

- Separate the wrists while pointing the index fingers downward.

## Gyana mudra

- Touch the base of your thumb with the tip of your index finger and keep the hands on your knees with palms facing down.

## Hriday mudra

- Touch the base of the thumbs with the tips of the index fingers of the respective hands.
- Join the tips of the thumbs with the tips of the middle and ring fingers.
- The little fingers should be away and straight.
- Keep the hands on the knees with the palms facing down.
- Hold the posture for 5 minutes.

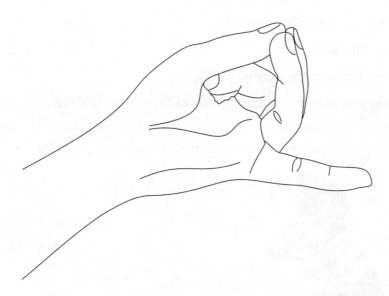

## Maha mudra

- Sit down with the legs stretched out in front of you.

- Bending the left leg, keep the left heel against the perineum.

- Fold the tongue back and inhale deeply.

- Exhaling, bend forward and hold the big toe with both the hands.

- Inhaling slowly in ujjayi, bend the head a little backwards.

- Concentrate on the space between the eyebrows and contract the perineum.

- Retaining the breath in, move your mind over the chakras from agnya to mooladhara; while repeating their names in the mind.

- Continue the repetition of names till comfortable.

- Relax the perineum and the eyes.

- Exhaling, bring your head back to the normal position.

- Repeat 3 times on either side and then 3 times with both legs stretched out in front.

*This mudra should not be done if you have heart ailments or when the blood is toxic.*

*Yoga and Diet for Ailments*

## Shajoli

- Sit in padmasana and bend your body a little forward.
- Inhale and retaining the breath in, contract your urethra, and hold it for a few seconds.
- Exhaling, release the contraction and relax for 2 to 3 seconds; then repeat.
- Practise 50 times.
- This mudra can be done faster without breath retention.

*This mudra should not be done if you have infection or inflammation of the urethra.*

## Sambhavi mudra

- Close your eyes and relax the body.
- Open your eyes and look up and focus your gaze on the point between the eyebrows.
- In the correct position, this part forms a 'V'.
- Gaze at the tip of the 'V' for a few seconds, and then close the eyes.
- Repeat 3 rounds; gradually increasing the duration of each round.

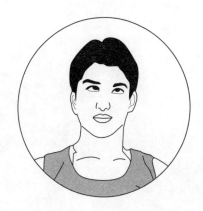

*This mudra should not be done if you have glaucoma, retinopathy or if you've recently had an eye surgery.*

## Shanmukhi mudra

- Sit in padmasana and plug your ears with the thumbs.
- Place the index fingers on your closed eyes.
- Close the nostrils with the middle fingers and keep the ring fingers under the nose.
- Keep the little fingers under the lips.
- Remove the middle fingers and breathe deeply.
- Close the nostril again and hold the breath for as long as comfortable.
- Exhale.
- Repeat for 2 to 3 minutes.

*This mudra should not be done if you have depression.*

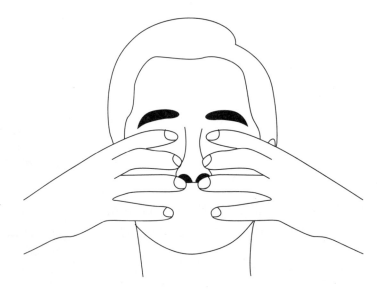

# BANDHA

## Jalandhara bandha

- Sit in padmasana with the hands on the knees.

- Take a deep breath.

- Holding the breath in, bend your head forward and press the chin to the chest.

- Lift the shoulders to straighten the arms, pressing the knees in the process.

- Hold the posture for as long as comfortable.

- Release the shoulder lock.

- Lift head up and breathe out.

- Repeat after a few seconds when the breathing is back to normal.

- Practise 5 times

*This bandha should not be done if you have heart ailments, high blood pressure, vertigo or cervical spondylitis.*

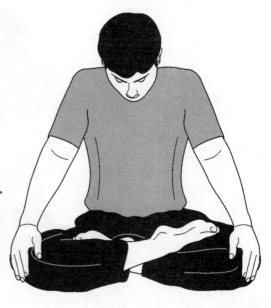

# Moola bandha

- Assume jalandhara bandha.
- Contract the perineum.
- Hold the posture till comfortable.
- Release the perineum; release shoulder lock and lift the head to normal position and inhale.
- Repeat 5 times.

*This bandha should not be done if you have heart ailments, high blood pressure, vertigo or cervical spondylitis.*

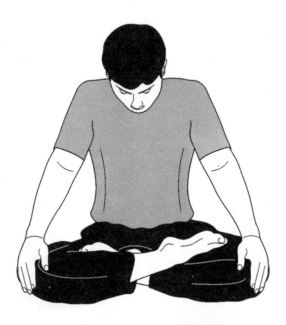

## Uddiyana bandha

- Sit in padmasana.

- Take a deep breath.

- Exhaling through pursed lips, making a hissing sound, drop the head to the chest to assume jalandhara bandha.

- Contract your stomach all the way to the spine.

- Hold this posture for as long as comfortable.

- Relax the stomach, release the shoulder lock and lift the head up and inhale.

- Wait till breathing is normal, then practise again.

- Repeat 5 times.

*This bandha should not be done if you have stomach ulcer, colitis, heart ailments, high blood pressure or glaucoma.*

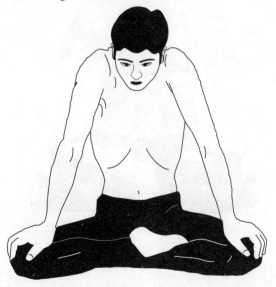

## Maha bandha

- This is a combination of all the three bandhas.

- Exhaling, assume jalandhara. Then contract the perineum and lastly pull the stomach in.

- While releasing the bandhas, do it first with the perineum, then the stomach, and lastly the shoulders.

*This bandha should not be done if you have any of the abovementioned diseases (related to the three bandhas).*

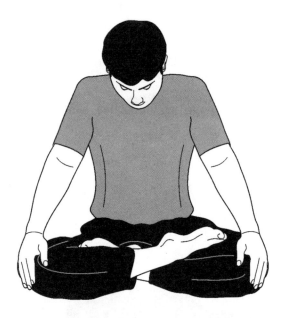

# 12

# Healing Recipes

## ALKALINE DIET

An alkaline diet a great way to guard health and prevent many diseases especially cancer. Most non-sour fruits and vegetables (in the raw form) are highly alkaline; and so are certain nuts and sprouts. But too much of raw vegetables can inhibit thyroxin production. And taking only fruit and nuts, although considered as one of the best food options, can cause problems in the long run. Therefore, to be on the safer side, one should not take a raw (fruits and vegetables) diet for more than three months at a stretch.

A strictly raw food diet should only be followed by cancer patients who need to alkalize their blood quickly. People with other acid related problems such as acidity, arthritis and gastritis can include non acidic or low acidic cooked food as well.

# ALKALINE DIET

## Some common foods that are acidic

- Underground vegetables except carrot. Other acidic vegetables are cauliflower, capsicum, lady's finger, brinjal, and pumpkin,

- All pulses except green gram

- Non-vegetarian food, non-fatty fish being the least acidic

- Most nuts except almond, walnut etc

- Leafy vegetables except lettuce, 'chaulai' 'bathua' coriander and mint

- Mustard, red chilli

- White flour

- Anything that tastes sour including citrus fruits. Melon, although tastes sweet is an acidic fruit.

- Coffee and black boiled tea


## A SAMPLE CHART OF ALKALINE DIET (the quantity can be adjusted)

### BREAKFAST

- 2 tablespoons each of green gram, fenugreek and alfalfa sprouts
- 1 banana
- 5 almonds

- 1 rose hip
- 1 amla
- 1 tablespoon blackstrap molasses
- 1 glass green juice (made from wheat grass, celery, basil, betel, and bel leaf i.e., wood apple)

## LUNCH

- Green coconut jelly
- 1 tablespoon each of black chick pea alfalfa and green gram sprouts
- 1 apple
- 1 carrot
- ½ cucumber
- Green coriander and mint chutney with green chili
- 1 bunch of grapes
- 1 guava
- 1 tablespoon blackstrap molasses
- 1 tablespoon coconut

## DINNER

- 1 banana
- 1 teaspoon blackstrap molasses
- 1 teaspoon honey
- 1-2 lettuce leaves
- 2 figs

*Yoga and Diet for Ailments*

- 2 dates
- 2-3 walnuts
- 1 teaspoon flaxseeds

## FORENOON

- Green tea with honey

## MORNING

- Petha (ash gourd) and lauki (bottle gourd) juice

## AFTERNOON

- Green coconut water

## EVENING

- Green tea with honey

## NEUTRAL AND LOW ACID RECIPES

In some recipes, you will need these 5 spices for tempering:

- 100 grams mustard seeds
- 50 grams cumin seeds
- 25 grams fenugreek
- 25 grams fennel
- 25 grams caraway seeds

Mix these 5 spices together and use it when needed.

# VEGETARIAN

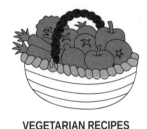

**VEGETARIAN RECIPES**

## Gourd Garlic

### Ingredients

500 grams bottle gourd

7-8 cloves of garlic

1 green chili

1 tablespoon cow's ghee or olive oil

Water (if necessary)

Salt to taste

### Method

Wash and peel the gourd and cut it into half inch cubes. Chop garlic and split the chili. Put the gourd in a pan, add salt and cover it. Cook on low heat. When vegetables begin to leave water, uncover the pan. Cook till soft and when all the water dries up, remove from heat and keep aside. Heat oil/ghee and fry the garlic till golden brown. Add chili and after 10-15 seconds, add the cooked vegetable along with water. After a minute or so remove from heat.

## Green Papaya with Curry Leaves

### Ingredients

500 grams green papaya

½ teaspoon mustard seeds

3-4 sprigs of curry leaves

1-2 teaspoon of ghee or oil

½ cup water

1-2 green chilies

Salt to taste

## Method

Wash, peel, and cube the papaya. Cook the vegetables with salt and water, till soft. Heat oil and add mustard seeds to it. When they start crackling, break the chilies and add them with the curry leaves. Pour in the vegetables along with its broth. Let it cook for a minute or so. Remove from heat.

## Zucchini Poppy Seeds

### Ingredients

500 grams zucchini

2 tablespoons poppy seeds

2 green chilies

¼ teaspoon caraway seeds

1 tablespoon oil or ghee

3-4 tablespoon water

Salt to taste

### Method

Wash and dice zucchini. Grind the poppy seeds and split the chilies. Cook the vegetables with water and salt till they are half done and almost dry. Add the poppy seeds to it and stir well. Remove from heat. In another pan, heat oil, and add caraway seeds and chilies to it. When the crackling stops, add the cooked vegetables and simmer. Cover and stir till dry and cooked.

## Papaya Poppy Seeds

### Ingredients

500 grams green papaya

1 medium onion

2 tablespoon poppy seeds

1 teaspoon coriander powder

½ teaspoon turmeric powder

1 bay leaf

1-2 green chili

1 small piece of cinnamon

1 tablespoon oil or ghee

½ cup water

Salt to taste

### Method

Wash, peel, and cube the papaya. Chop onions and slit green chilies. Grind the poppy seeds. Heat oil and add bay leaf to it. When its colour changes, add onion and fry till golden brown. Add turmeric powder, coriander powder, chili, salt, and fry for a minute. Add papaya and salt and fry for another minute. Pour water and cook till soft and almost dry. Remove from heat. Grind cinnamon with one tablespoon of water; pour over the curry and mix well.

## Ridge Gourd Curry

### Ingredients

500 grams ridge gourd

½ teaspoon 5 tempering spices

1 onion

7-8 cloves of garlic

1-2 green chilies

1 tablespoon oil or ghee

½ tsp turmeric powder

Salt to taste

### Method

Wash, peel, and slice vegetables in long strips. Chop onion and garlic. Split the chilies. Heat oil and add the 5 spices. As the spluttering subsides, add onion, garlic and chilies, and fry till the onion turns translucent. Add vegetables, salt, and turmeric powder and simmer till done.

## Broccoli Omum

### Ingredients

500 grams broccoli

¼ teaspoon omum seeds

4-5 tablespoon milk

2 tablespoon ghee or oil

Salt to taste

**Method**

Wash and chop the broccoli into big pieces. Heat oil. Add the omum seeds and after a seconds, add the broccoli. Fry on low heat for 2 to 3 minutes. Pour in the milk, add salt and simmer till cooked well.

## Broccoli Garlic

**Ingredients**

500 grams broccoli

1 pod garlic

½ cup water

Salt to taste

**Method**

Wash and chop the broccoli into small pieces. Heat oil, add chopped garlic and fry till golden brown and aromatic. Add broccoli and salt and fry on low heat for a minute. Pour water and cook till done. Make sure that the broccoli remains crunchy.

# Veg Stew

## Ingredients

200 grams peas

200 grams broccoli

200 grams carrot

½ coconut

1 bay leaf

1 black cardamom

10 peppercorns

½ cup water

2 teaspoon ghee or oil

Salt to taste

## Method

Shell peas. Wash and scrape carrots before dicing them. Chop broccoli into big pieces. Grate the coconut and extract its milk. Cook the vegetables with salt, water, cardamom, and peppercorn. After it is cooked properly, pour in the milk and let it simmer for 2 to 3 minutes. Keep aside.

In another pan, heat oil and add the bay leaf. When it starts to change its colour, pour it over the stew.

# NON-VEGETARIAN

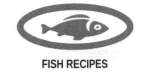

**FISH RECIPES**

## Fish Caraway

### Ingredients

4 pieces fish

½ turmeric powder

¼ teaspoon caraway seeds

6 cloves of garlic

1 green chilli

1 small onion

2 teaspoon cow's ghee, mustard oil or olive oil

1 cup water

Salt to taste

### Method

Wash the fish and smear it with turmeric powder. Chop onion and garlic and slit the chilli. Heat oil and add the caraway seeds. When they crackle, add the onion and garlic, and fry till they turn transparent. Pour in the water and let it boil for a while. Put the fish in the pan and reduce heat. Let it simmer till the fish is almost cooked. Add the chili and remove when done.

*Yoga and Diet for Ailments*

## Fish Coconut

**Ingredients**

4 pieces fish

½ coconut

½ onion

7-8 cloves of garlic

20-30 curry leaves

2 green chilies

A pinch of turmeric powder

2 teaspoon cow's ghee or olive oil

1 cup water

Salt to taste

**Method**

Wash fish and smear it with turmeric powder. Extract the coconut milk with ½ cup water. Chop the onion and garlic and split the green chillies. Mix all the ingredients and cook on low heat till done.

## Fish Poppy Seeds

**Ingredients**

4 pieces fish

1 tablespoon poppy seeds

1 tablespoon coconut

1 green chili

A pinch of turmeric powder

A sprig of mint leaves

1 teaspoon ghee or olive oil

1 teaspoon mustard oil

Salt to taste

**Method**

Wash the fish and let it dry. Marinate it with mustard oil and turmeric powder and set aside. Dry roast the poppy seeds, and coconut, and grind them with all the ingredients (except oil). Coat the fish pieces with this paste; Keep the fish pieces in a banana leaf or foil and steam for 7 to 8 minutes.

## Fish Curry

**Ingredients**

4 pieces fish

2 teaspoon cumin seeds

1 teaspoon coriander seeds

½ teaspoon turmeric powder

1 green chili

½ teaspoon 5 spices for tempering

2 teaspoon olive oil or cow's ghee

1 cup water

**Method**

Wash fish and smear it with turmeric. Grind cumin and coriander powder with water. Heat oil and put the 5 spices. When they crackle, put in the chili and the ground spices. Fry for 1 to 2 minutes. Add fish and fry for another minute or so. Add water and cook till done.

## Baked Fish

**Ingredients**

4 pieces fish

1 pod garlic

1 teaspoon ghee or oil

Salt to taste

**Method**

Wash and dry the fish. Grind the garlic coarsely. Mix all the spices and marinate the fish with it for 10 to 15 minutes. Bake it for 7 minutes on high temperature.

# Soya Fish

## Ingredients

4 pieces fish

2 tablespoon soya sauce

1 medium spring onion

6-7 cloves of garlic

½ green chili

1 teaspoon oil

1 bay leaf

¼ cup water

Salt to taste

## Method

Wash and dry the fish. Grind the garlic and chili, and chop the onion. Mix all the ingredients together and cook on low heat till it is almost dry.

# MEDICINAL RECIPES

## Garlic Toast

**Ingredients**

1 slice bread

20 cloves of garlic

1 tablespoon ghee or oil

**Method**

Chop garlic. Heat the ghee and fry the garlic in it. Remove and spread it on the bread. Grill till it turns a nice brown.

## Kadha for Cold

**Ingredients**

25 basil leaves

4 bay leaves

10 peppercorns

1 inch ginger

2 black cardamoms

1 glass of water

1 tablespoon honey

## Method

Boil all the ingredients (except honey) together till it evaporates to a quantity equal to one cup. Remove and let it cool for a little while. It should be hot, but not steaming hot. Mix the honey.

## Yogic Tea

### Ingredients

20 basil leaves

1 bay leaf

7 peppercorns

1" ginger

1 tsp tea leaves

Sugar to taste

1½ cup water

### Method

Crush ginger. Put all the ingredients together except tea leaves and boil till water is reduced to almost half. Add tea leaves, cover and leave it for 10 -15 seconds. Remove from fire.

## Coconut Oil

**Ingredients**

1 coconut

1½ cup of water

**Method**

Grate the coconut and pour half a cup of boiling water over it. Keep aside for half an hour. Strain out the coconut milk. Heat the rest of the water and repeat the process.

Heat the extracted coconut and let it boil till most of it evaporates. Turn down the flame and let it cook on very low heat. Wait till all the water dries up, leaving behind the oil.

## Oil for Cold

**Ingredients**

1 tablespoon mustard oil

½ teaspoon caraway seeds

5-6 cloves of garlic

**Method**

Add chopped garlic and caraway seeds to hot oil. Stir till the garlic is almost charred. Remove from fire; cool and store. Make sure that you do not store it for more than 2 to 3 days.

When you feel cold, warm this oil a little, and apply it on the soles.

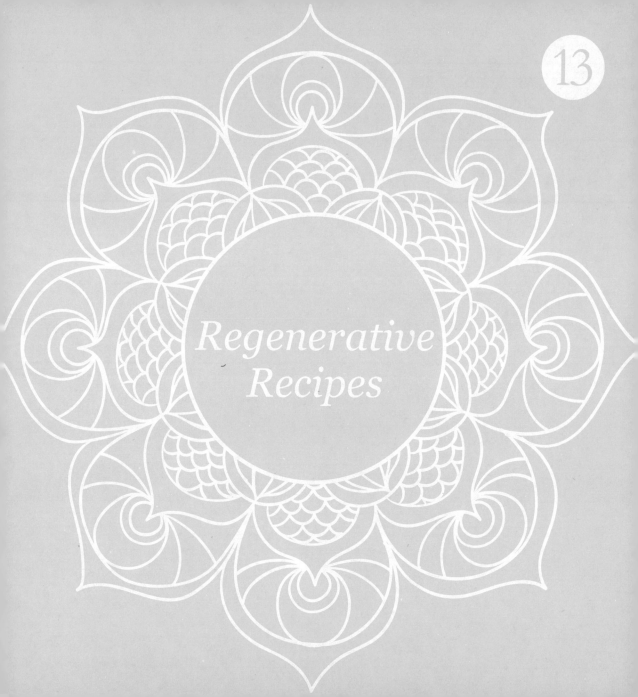

# 13

# Regenerative
# Recipes

Foods rich in nucleic acid help in the development of young and healthy cells. Nucleic acid is a special protein that is present in each cell, and it supervises the growth and multiplication of body tissues. The last two letters of DNA in fact stand for nucleic acid. If these acids get damaged due to free radicals or improper food, the information coded in the cells' DNA is distorted; which then leads to the reproduction of imperfect cells. This results in faster ageing and ill health. But, taking a diet rich in nucleic acid can make the system acidic. To prevent this, it is necessary to balance one's diet with strong alkaline food. The recipes in this chapter are devised accordingly.

# NON-VEGETARIAN

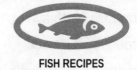

**FISH RECIPES**

## Sardine Aspargus

### Ingredients

200 grams sardine

1 onion

100 grams asparagus

1 carrot

2 tablespoon olive oil

Salt to taste

10-12 pepper corns

### Method

Cook the sardine in 1 tablespoon oil and half a cup of water, till it becomes soft and dry. Cut the asparagus and carrot into 3 inch long strips and blanch them. Chop onion coarsely. Crush pepper corns. Heat the rest of the oil and fry onion till translucent. Add vegetables and sauté for a minute. Add sardines and seasoning. Mix carefully before removing from heat.

## Prawns In Green

### Ingredients

250 grams prawns

100 grams bak choy

1 radish (with leaves)

100 grams lettuce

10-12 cloves of garlic

½ cup vegetable stock

1 tablespoon olive oil

Salt to taste

**Method**

Shell, de-vein, and wash the prawns. Cut the greens into big pieces. Chop garlic. Cut radish into small pieces. Heat oil in a wok. Add the garlic and fry for a few seconds. Add all the vegetables and fry until tender. Pour the stock and add salt. Cook till almost cooked. Put prawns and fry for 3 to 4 minutes and remove. Do not overcook the prawns as they might become hard.

## Sardine with Zucchini

**Ingredients**

200 grams sardine

1 zucchini

50 grams mushroom

2 onions

½ teaspoon crushed pepper

2 tablespoon olive oil

Salt to taste

*Yoga and Diet for Ailments*

## Method

Cook the sardine with 1 tablespoon oil and half a cup of water till the water evaporates and the fish becomes tender. Cut onion into thick slices. Dice mushroom and zucchini into big chunks, and blanch them. Heat the rest of the oil and put all the vegetables together and fry. When the vegetables are almost cooked, add the fish. Sprinkle pepper and stir well. Remove when cooked.

## Fish Rice

### Ingredients

200 grams sardine

2 cups cooked rice

1 onion

7-8 cloves of garlic

1 small beetroot

A pinch of nutmeg powder

1 to 2 green chilies

2 tablespoon oil

Salt to taste

### Method

Cook the sardine with 1 tablespoon oil and half a cup of water, till it becomes tender and dry. Cook, peel and dice the beetroot. Chop onion and garlic. Split the chilli lengthwise (you can chop it if you want it to be spicier). Heat oil and fry the onion till brown. Add garlic and sauté for a few seconds, before adding the beetroot and chilli. Fry for another minute or so and then add rice, nutmeg and salt. Fry for 2 to 3 minutes. Add the fish and mix well.

## Salmon Broccoli

### Ingredients

200 grams salmon

100 grams broccoli

10-12 cloves of garlic

1 tablespoon ghee (clarified butter)

Salt to taste

### Method

Wash and dry the fish. Chop broccoli into big pieces and blanch it. Peel and grind the garlic. Mix ghee, garlic, and salt; and apply it on the fish and broccoli. Marinate and keep aside for 10 minutes. Grill the fish for 7 minutes.

## Sea Bass and Cauliflower

### Ingredients

200 grams sea bass

200 grams cauliflower

1 big onion

½ teaspoon crushed pepper

A bunch of coriander leaves

1 tablespoon oil or ghee

Salt to taste

**Method**

Slice the fish into one inch pieces; sprinkle salt and keep aside. Chop the cauliflower into big pieces. Slice thick pieces of onion. Clean the coriander leaves and keep aside. Cook the cauliflower with salt in one fourth cup of water, until the water evaporates completely. In a wok, heat the oil/ghee till it smokes. Twirl the wok to coat all sides. Put the fish in the middle and the vegetables around it. Sprinkle pepper on top. After a minute, turn the fish and vegetables. Break the coriander leaves in half and spread all over. Turn once or twice again, before removing from fire.

## Sardine Gourd Sandwich

**Ingredients**

200 grams sardine

500 grams bottle gourd

A small bunch of mint leaves

A small bunch of coriander leaves

1 big onion

2 tablespoon ghee or oil

8 slices of whole wheat bread

1 tablespoon cider vinegar

Salt to taste

**Method**

Cook the fish in 1 tablespoon oil and half a cup of water, till the water evaporates, and the fish becomes tender. Grate gourd and cook it with salt. Grind coriander and mint leaves and add to the gourd. Add vinegar, salt, and chopped sardine to the bottle gourd mixture. Spread the mixture and an onion slice on the bread slices. Serve grilled.

# VEGETARIAN

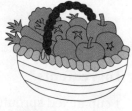

**VEGETARIAN RECIPES**

## Sprouts Sandwich

### Ingredients

1 tablespoon green gram sprouts

1 teaspoon black chick peas sprouts

1 teaspoon alfalfa sprouts

7 almonds

50 grams button mushroom

100 grams ash gourd or bottle gourd

2 slices whole wheat bread

2 slices rice bran bread

2 slices barley or rye bread

1 tablespoon olive oil

Salt and pepper to taste

### Method

Soak 7 almonds overnight. The next day, peel its skin and grind it with all the sprouts. Grate the gourd and chop the mushroom. Cook these vegetables with salt. Mix the vegetables and sprouts mixture. Add salt and pepper to taste. Spread the mixture on each bread slice (3 different types of breads). Stack together the 3 slices to make the sandwich. Cut the sandwich diagonally.

# Sprouts Pancake with Beet Chutney

## Ingredients

1 cup mixed sprouts

½ cup rice

400 grams cauliflower

300 grams coriander leaves

1 beetroot

2 tablespoon cider vinegar

1-2 green chilies

Ghee or olive oil

A pinch of red chili powder

Salt to taste

## Method

Soak rice for 5 to 6 hours. Grind it with the sprouts into a smooth batter. Keep aside.

**To make the filling:** Grate cauliflower. Chop coriander leaves. Split the chilli into 2 halves. Heat 1 tablespoon oil/ghee and fry the chili in it. Then slowly add the vegetables and salt. Cover and cook on low flame till the vegetables are half-cooked. Then uncover and cook until dry.

**To make pancakes:** Add salt and a pinch of chili powder to the batter. If necessary, add a little water. The batter should be thick and of pouring consistency. Heat a flat frying pan. Coat it nicely with a little oil. When hot, pour half a cup of batter, and spread it nicely (around 0.25 inch thick). When one side is cooked, turn the pancake gently and cook the other side as well. Spread the filling on the pancake and roll it. Remove from fire and serve it with chutney.

**To make chutney:** Pressure cook the beetroot. Peel and grind it. Mix vinegar, salt, and a little red chilli powder; and serve with the pancakes.

## Zucchini Mushroom Sprouts

### Ingredients

200 grams zucchini

100 grams mushroom

½ cup green gram sprouts

7 almonds

7-8 cloves of garlic

1 tablespoon ghee or olive oil

Salt to taste

### Method

Cut zucchini into 1 inch chunks and dice the mushrooms. Fry almonds in a little oil. Heat oil/ghee and fry chopped garlic in it. Add vegetables and sauté. Add salt and reduce heat. Cover and cook till done. Add the sprouts and stir for a minute or two. Pound the nuts coarsely and sprinkle on top.

## Sprouts Chaat

### Ingredients

½ cup mixed sprouts

1 bunch coriander leaves

¼ onion

Puffed rice

1 tablespoon roasted peanuts

Chaat masala

Salt and chili powder to taste

### Method

Chop onion and coriander leaves, and mix it with the sprouts. Sprinkle puffed rice and peanuts on top and add seasonings as per taste.

---

## Sprouts Cutlet

### Ingredients

Cabbage

Green gram sprouts

1 onion

1 green chili

A small bunch of coriander leaves

½ teaspoon coriander powder

1 slice brown bread

¼ teaspoon garam masala

Salt to taste

Oil for shallow frying

**Method**

Shred cabbage and pressure cook with salt. Strain water and let it cool. Chop chili, onion, and coriander leaves. Soak bread in water for half an hour. Grind the sprouts coarsely. Squeeze water from the bread and mix it with sprouts, cabbage, onion, chili, coriander leaves, spices, and salt. Shape cutlets and shallow fry. Serve cutlets with apple chutney.

## Apple Chutney

**Ingredients**

½ apple

8-10 cloves of garlic

1 tablespoon cider vinegar

A small bunch of mint leaves

1 or ½ green chilli

Salt to taste

**Method**

Grind all the ingredients into a paste and serve it with cutlets.

# Mushroom Cauliflower Rice

## Ingredients

½ cup rice

100 grams mushroom

200 grams cauliflower

7-8 cloves of garlic

1-2 green chilies

1 tablespoon ghee or olive oil

1 cup water

Salt to taste

## Method

Dice vegetables and chop garlic. Wash and drain rice. Heat oil and fry garlic for a few seconds. Add mushrooms and cauliflowers, and sauté for a minute or so. Add rice; mix well and fry for a minute. Add water, salt and chilies, and pressure cook till cooked. Serve rice with green chutney.

# Green Chutney

## Ingredients

1 small bunch mint leaves

1 small bunch coriander leaves

4-5 leaves of lettuce

2 tablespoon cider vinegar

1 teaspoon jaggery

1 green chili

½ teaspoon cumin seeds

½ inch ginger

A pinch of black salt (optional)

Salt to taste

**Method**

Grind all the ingredients into a paste.

## Sprouts Curry

**Ingredients**

½ cup green gram sprouts

Cauliflower

Green papaya

Any gourd

Cumin seeds

½ inch ginger

1 red chili

1 tablespoon ghee

1 cup water

Salt to taste

## Method

Dice vegetables into big chunks. Crush ginger. Dry roast cumin and red chilli till brown, and keep aside. Fry sprouts in ghee till aromatic. Add water, vegetables, salt and ginger, and pressure cook till cooked. Sprinkle the dry roasted powder and serve with steamed rice.

# References

Kristine M. Napier, *Eat to Heal*, Warner Books. 1998

Ann Wigmore, *Be Your Own Doctor*, Avery Publisher Group. 2nd Edition 1983.

Dr. Michael Sharon, *Nutrients A to Z*, Prion Books. 2004

Dr. Aman, *Medicinal Secrets of Your Food.*

J. D. Ritcliff, *I am Joe's Body*, Berkley Publishing Group, New York. 1982.

David E. Larson, *Mayo Clinic Family Health Book*, William Morrow & Company, Inc., New York. 1990.

7. Ernest R. Hilgard, Rita L. Atkinson and Richard C. Atkinson, *Introduction to Psychology*, Harcourt Brace Jovanorich Inc. 1979.

Robert A. Baron, *Psychology*, Prentice Hall College Division, 4th Edition. 1999.

Jose Silva and Philip Miele, *The Silva Mind Control Method*, Pocket Books. 1991.

Jose Silva with Robert B. Stone, *The Silva Mind Control Method for Getting Help from Your Other Side*, Pocket Books. 1989.

Swami Sivananda, *Health and Hygiene*, Divine Life Society. 6th Edition 1996.

Swami Sivananda, *Japa Yoga*, Divine Life Society. 11th Edition 1994.

Swami Sivananda, *Mind – Its Mysteries and Control*, Divine Life Society. 12th Edition 1994.

Swami Sivananda, *Sure Ways for Success in Life & God Realization*, Divine Life Society. 13th Edition 1990.

Swami Sivananda, *Concentration and Meditation*, Divine Life Society. 8th Edition 1990.

Yogi Ramacharaka, *Hatha Yoga*, Kessinger Publishing. 1998.

Yogi Ramacharaka, *Fourteen Lessons in Yogi Philosophy and Oriental Occultism*, Kessinger Publishing. 2003.

Paramahamsa Yogananda, *Autobiography of a Yogi*, Self Realisation Fellowship Publisher. 1979.

*Hatha Yoga Pradipika*, Bihar School of Yoga, Munger. 1985.

Swami Satyananda Saraswati, *Asana Pranayama Mudra Bandha*, Bihar School of Yoga, Munger. 2nd Edition 1971.

Swami Satyananda Saraswati, *Yoga Nidra*, Bihar School of Yoga, Munger.

Swami Satyananda Saraswati, *Meditation from Tantra*, Bihar School of Yoga, Munger. 5th Edition 1983.

Swami Satyananda Saraswati, *Self Realisation*, Bihar School of Yoga, Munger.

Swami Satyananda Saraswati, *Yogic Cure for Common Diseases*, Bihar School of Yoga, Munger. 1983.

*Teaching of Swami Satyananda Saraswati*, Bihar School of Yoga. Vol. I First Australian Edition 1981, Vol. IV 4th Enlarged Edition 1986 & Vol. V 1986.

Visnu Devananda, *Meditation and Mantras*.

Choa Kok Sui, *The Ancient Science & Art of Pranic Healing*, Institute for Inner Studies. 1987.

Swami Muktananda Saraswati, *Nawayogini Tantra*. 1975.

Swami Satyananda Saraswati, *Yoga Education for Children*. 1985.

# Index of Practices

*Yoga and Diet for Ailments*

# Index of Recipes

Disclaimer:

Yoga is a practical science which should be learnt directly from an expert who can choose the practices according to the practitioner's physical and mental condition. An unsuitable regime followed incorrectly can lead to adverse consequences. The author shall not take any responsibility for such eventualities.

Improvement depends on the age and conditions of the practitioner.